'Bold, new/old terms, diffraction, new n
blages, interconnected becomings, and r
autobiographical, lyrical, standing on the
Guattari, Bronwyn's new book leads us ir

Norman K. D ... Professor of Sociology,
University of Illinois Urbana–Champaign

'In *Entanglement in the World's Becoming and the Doing of New Materialist Inquiry*, Bronwyn Davies has written an unputdownable page-turner. It is a rare and exciting scholarly text that draws readers in. This is a clear, beautifully written book that deserves more than one reading. The writing is powerful, vulnerable and absorbing. This work is written with the generosity and sympathy that it offers and advocates. It is a book that deserves, and evokes, our attention and response-ability'.

Jane Speedy, Emeritus Professor of Education, University of Bristol

'*Entanglement in the World's Becoming and the Doing of New Materialist Inquiry* is a lucid, engrossing and energising, deep dive into the possibilities and challenges facing qualitative researchers in these times. Bronwyn Davies takes us through the implications of theory into a series of experimental forays into life itself, where the researcher is implicated at every turn. This is a turn to 'ambulatory' methods and modes of thought: expansive, creative, unsettling and thrilling. She develops new areas of inquiry and revisits classic work on gender, subjectivity, children, schooling, academic life, intimacy, abjection, recognition, the body in place by entering into potent and often poignant moments of being and becoming. Anyone who has ever read and loved her work will be stunned again by the freshness of her thinking, rigorous and clear-eyed theoretical engagement, and courageous recasting of what it might be to be a researcher entangling with the world'.

Susanne Gannon, Associate Professor of Education,
Western Sydney University

'Once again, Bronwyn Davies has written a tantalising guide to the possibilities of research that entangle new materialist philosophy with post-qualitative research, autoethnography and collective biography, though this time the project is further enhanced by its engagement with the visual arts and literature. Each central chapter provides a different exemplar that works through entanglements that draw on aspects of family history, gendered violence, the position of children in the world, indigenous recognition and/or vibrant life beyond narrow definitions of the human. Each exemplar could stand alone as an inspiring guide for researchers seeking new approaches, but again Davies takes this further with final reflections on the pressing implications for life entangled within a global pandemic. At times intensely personal, the complex yet beautifully written texts go beyond the specificities of individual experience to give space for the re-vitalising insights that new materialist analyses can offer, while also raising questions about ethical "response-abilities" that call to us now from the present and the past'.

Lise Claiborne, Adjunct Professor of Education,
University of Waikato

'Bronwyn Davies has an extraordinary talent for doing justice to theoretical complexity while at the same time bringing that complexity accessibly to life. The reader can't help but learn. The reader can't help but be affected. Those of us seeking to draw upon the new materialisms in our research and writing are deeply in her debt'.

Jonathan Wyatt, Professor of Qualitative Inquiry,
The University of Edinburgh

'When beginning my journey into 'thinking differently' and post-structuralism, I wondered why the language needed to be so difficult to understand and 'translate'. Bronwyn told me it was so that we did not slip into 'thinking as usual'. This book is certainly not thinking as usual when delving into new materialism. It takes us on a journey of moving beyond the already known, and calls us as researchers to find joy in being open to the not-yet-known. This is a world away from the current expectations most researchers experience in universities.

Bronwyn states that to do new materialist research is to find very different research questions that do not envisage humanity's existence as independent of, and separate from, the nonhuman or more-than-human world. This book takes us on a journey of being open to different research methodology – including *diffractive methodology, transcendental empiricism, and collective biography.* Each chapter talks us through how these might be done, then shows us these in action. At the end, and throughout, in each chapter, new materialist research is undertaken on the everyday – in the park, a pond, friendship, children, spaces, places, art, death, at home, swimming, on a train, under a tree.

Throughout the book Bronwyn explores the conception of new materialist ethics. "In place of the institutional ethics that tie down the research event to controlled and predictable practices and outcomes, new materialist ethics, in its unpredictability, never lets the researcher off the hook of considering how their emergent thoughts and actions matter". There is freedom and responsibilities of seeing ethics in this way.

The book speaks to me about research possibilities and while each chapter grows from another, the chapters *The Three Components of the Refrain* and *Recognition* I found the most exciting. New possibilities – lines of flight – are opened to me. I have no doubt each researcher will find the possibilities that open for them'.

Dr Cath Laws, Australian Catholic University

'This book demonstrates how new materialist concepts can be applied not only to research, but to relationship and workplace problems. Bronwyn shows how new concepts can help us arrive at very different conclusions about ourselves, others, and life, when we find ourselves in seemingly hopeless and frustrating situations. This book is very relevant for teachers and counsellors working in schools'.

Maria Kecskemeti PhD, Teacher and Counsellor, Wellington, New Zealand

ENTANGLEMENT IN THE WORLD'S BECOMING AND THE DOING OF NEW MATERIALIST INQUIRY

Entanglement in the World's Becoming and the Doing of New Materialist Inquiry explores new materialist concepts and the ways in which they provoke an opening up of thought about being human, and about being more-than-human. The more-than-human refers, here, to the world that we are of – a world that includes humans, who are emergent and permeable, and all of the animal and earth others they intra-act with. It explores how we affect those others and are affected.

This book engages intimately in encounters of various kinds, some drawn from the author's everyday life, some from the research projects she has engaged in over several decades, and some from others' research. It works at the interface of living- and writing-as-inquiry, delving into the rich seam of conceptual possibilities opened up by Deleuze and Guattari, and Barad, and by new materialist inquiry more broadly. It brings not just words to the task, but also art, photographs, movement, memories, bodies, sound, touch, things.

It delves into the ways in which the entangled dynamics of social, material and semiotic flows and forces make up the diffractive movements through which life emerges, assembles itself, and endures. New materialist concepts, as they are explored here, offer new and emergent approaches to life itself, and to ways in which we might research our lives as they are intricately enfolded in the life of the earth.

Bronwyn Davies is an independent scholar, with honorary professorships at the universities of Melbourne and Western Sydney. She left academe in protest ten years ago at the growing stranglehold of neoliberalism on academic work. She has written her best work since then and enjoyed several wonderful academic collaborations. See bronwyndavies.com.au for details.

ENTANGLEMENT IN THE WORLD'S BECOMING AND THE DOING OF NEW MATERIALIST INQUIRY

Bronwyn Davies

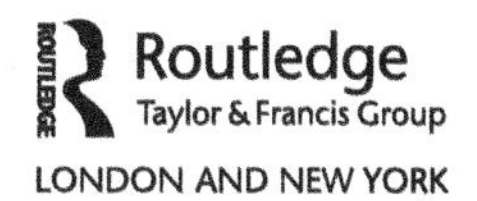

LONDON AND NEW YORK

First published 2021
by Routledge
2 Park Square, Milton Park, Abingdon, Oxon OX14 4RN

and by Routledge
52 Vanderbilt Avenue, New York, NY 10017

Routledge is an imprint of the Taylor & Francis Group, an informa business

British Library Cataloguing-in-Publication Data
A catalogue record for this book is available from the British Library

Library of Congress Cataloging-in-Publication Data
Names: Davies, Bronwyn, author.
Title: Entanglement in the world's becoming and the doing of new materialist inquiry / Bronwyn Davies.
Description: New York : Routledge, 2021. | Includes bibliographical references and index. |
Identifiers: LCCN 2020038204 (print) | LCCN 2020038205 (ebook) | ISBN 9780367479749 (hardback) | ISBN 9780367479756 (paperback) | ISBN 9781003037477 (ebook)
Subjects: LCSH: Social sciences--Research. | Social sciences--Philosophy. | Materialism. | Aesthetics. | Philosophy, Modern--21st century.
Classification: LCC H62 .D25428 2021 (print) | LCC H62 (ebook) | DDC 300.1--dc23
LC record available at https://lccn.loc.gov/2020038204
LC ebook record available at https://lccn.loc.gov/2020038205

ISBN: 978-0-367-47974-9 (hbk)
ISBN: 978-0-367-47975-6 (pbk)
ISBN: 978-1-003-03747-7 (ebk)

Typeset in Bembo
by SPi Global, India

CONTENTS

FIGURES

ACKNOWLEDGEMENTS

I began this book project with the question: what is it to be human? What do we really mean when we use terms such as posthuman and nonhuman and inhuman? Is our use of new materialist concepts just a conceptual game, or can it change the way we live and the way we do our research? Are these new concepts no more than stones thrown into a pond, sending out overlapping ripples on the water's surface then sinking to the bottom? Or are they more lively than that? What work do they do, *can* they do, to disrupt the seemingly intractable hierarchy that separates the dominant, individualised, neoliberalised human from its subordinated others? In what way do they change what it is to be human? In what way do they change how it is we might conduct our research? What are we to become in the process of mobilising these concepts in our lives and in our research practices? What are the ethical implications of taking up such powerful conceptual tools?

Part way through this project, out-of-control fires, the like of which had never been seen, started burning up the world along the east and south coasts of Australia, killing billions of animal and earth others, and destroying homes, and lives and livelihoods. The world that we are of was clearly in deep trouble, yet politicians were stubbornly, obtusely impervious to the stark and terrifying evidence of the need for radical change. Hot on the heels of that five-month conflagration was the coronavirus pandemic.

This book therefore had no chance of becoming a mild intellectual exercise. It has become, rather, a passionate exploration of life, not just of the intellect, but of the senses, of life that asks urgent questions of itself and of its response-ability to the world.

New materialism crosses disciplinary borders – individuals are no longer separate from the social, cultural and material world; and things matter. Thinking and feeling are not two separate processes. Binaries such as animate and inanimate can no longer hold as hierarchical opposites. And the past is not finished with, diffracting as it does with the present and the future. New materialist inquiry seeks life in its fullest possible expression, and it works toward new ways of thinking-doing creative-relational inquiry. Life is understood as its capacity to respond – its response-ability.

That response-ability is constitutive of this work. I could not have done this thinking and writing alone, independent of friends, family and colleagues, or independent of the matter of the Earth and its multiple forms of life. According to new materialist thought, I am of the world rather than in it, and in that sense this book is emergent from the world, rather than emergent from me as sole author. I acknowledge that world and the life it enables – a life I find utterly extraordinary.

Within that world are wonderful friends and colleagues: Peter Bansel, Lise Claiborne, Elisabeth de Schauwer, Susanne Gannon, Maria Kecskemeti, Cath Laws, Sheridan Linnell, Margaret Somerville, Jane Speedy, Jody Thomson, Geert van Hove, Jonathan Wyatt and Johanna Wyn, among many others. I am indebted to each of them for the conversations we have had, in which life always emerges as something new, and I am indebted to them for their sympathetic engagement with my thinking, writing and image-making. I am indebted to Norm Denzin for his support of my work, and for his *International Congress of Qualitative Inquiry*, which provides a space in which difference flourishes, and creative-relationality emerges. My thanks, too, to Hannah Shakespeare for inviting me to write this book, and for her unfailing support throughout.

Thanks to Jody Thomson for her drawing of Princess Barbie. Thanks to Bloomsbury Academic for permission to use excerpts from my chapter published as: Davies, B. (2020) Pondering the pond. Ethical encounters with children. In C. Schulte (ed.), *Ethical Encounters with Children: New Perspectives*. London: Bloomsbury Academic. Thanks to the Art Gallery of New South Wales and to Helen Brack for permission to print John Brack's *The New House* (Figure 8.5), and to the Art Gallery of New South Wales for permission to print Girolamo Nerli's *The Voyagers* (Figure 8.3). Thanks to Belinda Turner for her stunning photograph (Figure 5.1). I hope you see that I've used it, Belinda, and contact me so we can arrange a copyright payment.

Finally, I dedicate this book, with love, to my three sons, Paul, Jake and Dan, and my grandchildren, Ryan, Edie, Sam, Oscar, Gracie, Eric and Fred.

BRONWYN DAVIES

1

DELVING INTO NEW MATERIALISM

In which I introduce the reader to new materialist thought and practice, drawing in particular on Bergson, Deleuze and Barad. Some of the concepts I mobilise include intra-action, assemblage, lines of descent and ascent, ethico-onto-epistemology, diffraction, encounter and materiality. I discuss St Pierre's recommendation that we abandon method and I propose alternative ways of thinking and doing research inspired by new materialist concepts. I explore writing as inquiry with a poem about grief and letting go.

In this book I explore new materialist concepts and the ways they open up thought about being human, and about being more-than-human, where more-than-human refers to the world that we are of – a world that includes the emergent, permeable human and all of its animal and earth intra-active others. I carry out that exploration through encounters of various kinds that are drawn from my everyday life and from my own research, and sometimes the research of others. I work at the interface of living- and writing-as-inquiry, delving into the rich seam of conceptual possibilities opened up by Deleuze, Barad, and new materialist inquiry more broadly. I bring not just words to the task, but also art, photos, movement, memories, bodies, sound, touch, things...

New materialisms bring *ethics, ontology and epistemology* together in such a way that the concept-matter mix is never free of questions of responsibility and response-ability. Being is relational and never fixed; our responses matter; they have material affects and effects. Discourse and bodies affect each other, not in the sense of one shaping the other, but in *intra-action*; discourse and materiality each contribute to the conditions of possibility of the other: "the material and the discursive are mutually implicated in the dynamics of intra-activity" (Barad, 2003: 812), and each "assemblage, in its multiplicity, necessarily acts on semiotic flows, material flows, and social flows simultaneously" (Deleuze and Guattari, 1987: 22–23).

The entangled dynamics of social, material and semiotic flows and forces make up the diffractive movements through which life emerges, assembles itself, and endures. That capacity to endure depends on invention and creativity: "duration means invention, the creation of forms, the continual elaboration of the absolutely new" (Bergson, 1998: 11). At the same time, and this is important, *invention and creativity do not exist independent of the repetitions and rituals that make up much of everyday life*. They are inseparable from it:

> [I]n the universe itself two opposite movements are to be distinguished ... The first [descent] only unwinds a roll ready prepared. In principle, it might be accomplished almost instantaneously, like releasing a spring. But the ascending movement, which corresponds to an inner work of ripening or creating, *endures* essentially, and imposes its rhythm on the first, which is inseparable from it.
>
> (Bergson, 1998: 11)

Not one or the other, ascent *or* descent, with one dominant and the other subordinate, but an inter-dependent, intra-active relationship between the predictable (the movement of descent) and the new (the movement of ascent). Throughout this book I will come back to these opposing but inseparable movements, exploring them as they intra-act with each other, and as they contribute (or not) to life's capacity to endure.

Movement, then, is everywhere, even where we imagine there is none. Take, for example, a snowflake – an ice crystal, which looks rigid and frozen in place: "in reality, on an extremely tiny level, smaller than a couple of nanometers, as it freezes it vibrates like crazy, all the billion billion molecules that make it up shaking invisibly, practically burning up ... [and] tiny instabilities in those vibrations give snowflakes their individual shapes" (Doerr, 2005: 24).

> *Even the smallest bits of matter are an unfathomable multitude*
>
> (Barad, 2015: 160; emphasis added).

The poetics of living- and writing-as-inquiry

Living- and writing-as-inquiry is peculiarly suited to new materialisms (Wyatt, 2019; Wyatt et al., 2011). "Radical and provocative, disruptive and generative, writing-as-inquiry continues to open both itself and ourselves as qualitative scholars to new possibilities as we respond to the calls and challenges at the theoretical, methodological, ethical and political edges" (Wyatt, 2019: 7). It "reaches out beyond us, reaches in to where we may not want to go, a 'minor gesture' towards that which we do not know, to that which is beyond us" (Wyatt, 2019: 42).

Like the matter of the world, which is in constant motion, researchers, being *of* the world, are also in motion. They come to know the world through intra-actively engaging with it – that is, in each encounter they affect the world and are affected by it. And because ontology and epistemology are inseparable, epistemology can no longer be the sole medium through which the researcher thinks and does research.

We can no longer rely on what were once the reliable cornerstones of good research – the observation of a world that was rigorously separated from oneself, along with the taken-for-granted reliance on rational argument. New materialist researchers are epistemologically and ontologically integral to a world that is, in its most minute detail, intra-active; that is, they affect what they encounter, and are affected by it – they effect change, however minute, and are changed.

That mutual impact and indebtedness provides the conditions of possibility for a life: "'*Individuals' are infinitely indebted to all others, where indebtedness is not a debt that follows or results from a transaction but, rather, a debt that is the condition of possibility of giving/receiving*" (Barad, 2015: 160; emphasis added).

Concepts generated by new materialist scholars intra-act with the bodily matter of the researcher and with the matter and mattering being researched. New materialist researchers need strategies for inventing; they work with concepts, with words and ideas, and with multiple art forms that mobilise the senses. That invention, and the elaboration of the new, in Bergson's (1998) words, involves an inner work of ripening or creating, or creative evolution.

Generating the linguistic and material forms through which new thought can emerge, means breaking loose from habituated forms of research writing; it means searching for quite different linguistic and artistic forms of expression, and it means generating different ways of living life itself:

> [It means] striving to find inspiration in the arts, in the poetics of embodied living, in enacting the very un-actualized expressive and impressive potentials of social-scientific knowledge, in taking dedicated risks, in exercising passion, and in finding ways to re-configure thinking, sensing, and presenting by emphasizing the singular powers of action, locution, and thought.
>
> (Vannini, 2015: 319)

And I would add *intra-action* to Vannini's "action, locution and thought", in order to draw attention to the fact that we take up our existence in relation to others, to more-than-human others, to the organic and inorganic, to the epistemological and ontological.

Our capacity to affect others depends on an equal capacity to be affected. I use the term more-than-human here to include both animals and humans. Massumi plays across what were once clear borders between human and animal: "It is in becoming animal that the human recurs to what is nonhuman at the heart of what moves it. This makes it surpassingly human. Creative-relationally *more-than* human" (Massumi, 2015:14). I will be playfully stretching that *more-than* to include things like trees, ponds and artworks, as well as things like toys and watches and black velvet skirts.

Inquiry is necessarily never carried out alone. Writers write to and for readers. They are affected by those readers, as well as by other writers, by the material tools they work with, the material/emotional spaces they work in, and the geopolitical space–times that make such writing thinkable and do-able. In new materialist inquiry *the powers of action, intra-action, locution and thought are intimately entangled*: they affect each other; they are *emergent* in lines of ascent and descent; and they are integral to invention. Worked together, these powers offer new ways of thinking and doing research and writing.

The problem of method

St Pierre recommends that we abandon those established methods that tell us the correct way to do research, and that we immerse ourselves in reading, "reading and reading to find new concepts for thinking differently and then differently again" (2019: 13). We should trust ourselves, in Derrida's words, to begin "*wherever we are*; in a text where we already believe ourselves to be" (St Pierre, 2019: 12).

But abandoning familiar methods and beginning with oneself, is not without danger. Deleuze and Guattari warn against too radical an abandonment of the familiar in the search for the new:

> if you blow apart the strata without taking precautions, then instead of drawing the plane you will be killed, plunged into a black hole, or even dragged toward catastrophe. Staying stratified – organized, signified, subjected – is not the worst that can happen; the worst that can happen is if you throw the strata into demented or suicidal collapse, which brings them back down on us heavier than ever.
>
> (Deleuze and Guattari, 1987: 161)

Beginning where we are already has dual risks, on the one hand of being caught up in dominant tropes that rule out passion and poetics and the concept-matter mix, and on the other, of running us aground on the shoals of narcissism, creating the illusion that it is "all about me". Further, the petty bureaucratic practices of the institutions we work in can mean that "where we are at" is a place of conformity to the way things are done – which specifically excludes new forms of writing–thinking–being. Some Australian universities, for example, recently refused to recognise as research some of the chapters of the book *Writing with Deleuze in the Academy: Creating Monsters* (Riddle et al., 2018), on the grounds that the book challenges and disrupts the already-known, normative definitions of research. Research bureaucrats wielding official definitions of "research" concluded that the authors could have no credit for their work. In effect, the authors' lines of ascent were shut down by members of their institutions, administrative members, that is, who had themselves quite possibly never engaged in research. In the interests of neoliberal forms of productivity, and of preserving the academy as it is, the authors of *Writing with Deleuze* were refused the recognition they depend on to endure within the academy. The power of institutional assemblages to insist that there will be no new way of thinking and doing, can be formidable.

New materialism runs against the grain of neoliberal individualism and narcissism, which we have all been affected and infected by since the 1990s – and it runs against the grain of the centuries of liberal humanism and enlightenment thinking that have intimately informed our everyday lives. Our well-practised ways of lodging ourselves in the world may run counter to the new materialist challenge to encounter/encompass ourselves as a part of, and party to, multiple, dynamic life-worlds. We are inevitably caught in opposing flows or forces: we depend on our sense of ourselves as beings with specificity, even while we open ourselves to the interconnected becomings that will enable us to find ways to comprehend our own, and others', entanglement in the material world. Grosz describes the challenge of new materialist research this way:

> How can we produce knowledges, techniques, methods, practices that bring out the best in ourselves, that enable us to overcome ourselves, that open us up to the embrace of an unknown and open-ended future, that bring into existence new kinds of beings, new kinds of subjects, and new relations to objects?
> (2011: 75)

So, the question, I will suggest, is not so much one of whether we should do away with method and simply launch ourselves into life following extensive reading. I agree with St. Pierre that we don't need a prescriptive method, where the following of rules is imagined to guarantee some form of truth. What I want to explore here are approaches to methodology in which thinking and doing are intimately entangled, where they intra-act, and where invention and creativity impose their rhythms on the rituals and repetitions.

Methodology that responds to new materialist concepts addresses such questions as:

- How might we work with the material and emotional specificity of being human, entangled as being-human is with the more-than-human, while engaging with new concepts – concepts that open us up to the porous, collective, intra-active multiplicity of life?
- What encounters, what sympathies, what conceptual possibilities will dislodge habituated thoughts and practices, opening us up to new becomings and new ways of thinking-in-being, new ways of writing and researching – upending old habits of thought and practice, yet without too wildly destratifying?

To do new materialist research is to find very different research questions that do not envisage humanity's existence as independent of, and separate from, the nonhuman or more-than-human world. It involves asking, throughout the research process: in what ways can we become more responsible/response-able in our encounters with the human and with the more-than-human world, while not setting ourselves above or apart from it? It asks: how are we to engage in thinking and doing things differently? Bright puts the question in this way, as a conceptual problem to be lived with, and worked through:

> Here is a problem, then: to write to become someone other than who one is, to trace a line of becoming, when writing is thinking, and thinking is the

> engendering of thinking in thought. To resist a thought which pre-exists, interfering with practices, and disrupting the desire to erect a new façade over the ruins of humanism ... Making things happen, in other words. Making thinking happen.
>
> (Bright, 2018: 103–104)

A new materialist methodology does not provide a template. Adopting a ready-made set of practices and preconceived rules is antithetical to *any* good research (Davies and Gannon, 2006), and it is antithetical to the creative, experimental work that new materialism inspires. This does not mean research should be disorderly or undisciplined, but that it must remain open to the unexpected, to serendipity, and to new ways of thinking and doing as particular research questions and explorations take shape.

Diffraction: a material-discursive methodology

In a diffractive relationship "'each of us' is part of the intra-active ongoing articulation of the world in its differential mattering" (Barad, 2008: 333):

> The phenomenon of diffraction does not merely signify the disruption of representationalism and its metaphors of reflection in the endless play of images and its anxieties about copy and original and displacements of the Same elsewhere. Diffraction is an ethico-onto-epistemological matter. We are not merely differently situated in the world; "each of us" is part of the intra-active ongoing articulation of the world in its differential mattering. Diffraction is a material-discursive phenomenon that challenges the presumed inherent separability of subject and object, nature and culture, fact and value, human and nonhuman, organic and inorganic, epistemology and ontology, and material and discursive.
>
> (Barad, 2008: 332–333)

And, as Haraway says, seeing and thinking diffractively is about making a difference in the world: "What we need is to make a difference in material-semiotic apparatuses ... so that we get more promising interference patterns on the recording films of our lives and bodies" (1997: 16). She continues, explaining how diffraction works differently from reflection, a metaphor and practice that has the problem of an imagined original that can be copied. In contrast, "Diffraction patterns record the history of interaction, interference, reinforcement, difference. Diffraction is about heterogeneous history, not about originals ... Diffraction is a narrative, graphic, psychological, spiritual, and political technology for making consequential meanings" (Haraway, 1997: 273).

What I will do, throughout this book, is take you with me on multiple experimental forays, where I explore some of the diffractive forces – material, locutionary, ethical – that are at play. Such forays, in which new thought becomes possible, cannot always be planned ahead or controlled. We depend on chance, and on provocations that force us to think against the grain of our comfortable, safe repetitions. Being forced to think is not always comfortable. It's much easier and safer to let one's mind run along the well-worn tracks of the already known (Deleuze, 2000).

The diffractive methodologies of new materialism may sometimes be confronting, and they may seem too risky, yet they are almost always exciting in so far as they provoke new ways of thinking, new ways of being – new ways of *thinking-in-being*.

Sympoiesis, the collective creation of life, arises in multi-layered, intra-active encounters. *And because life itself is in motion, the truths we discover are fragile, no matter how carefully we document them*: "Ontological indeterminacy, a radical openness, an infinity of possibilities, is at the core of mattering ... Matter in its iterative materialisation is a dynamic play of in/determinacy. Matter is never a settled matter. It is always already radically open" (Barad, 2015: 160).

Through writing my way into a variety of encounters, I will explore the diffractive forces that impact on and emanate from human subjects, and more-than-human subjects, subjects who are *of* the world rather than *in* the world – subjects whose meanings reveal themselves, or whose meanings disappear in other realms, and might appear again quite changed. Not just writing, I hasten to add – images, works of art, the earth, the fire, the sun, the time of day, the wind, the wave, can be more powerful than words. The world with all its intricacies, its repetitions and lines of flight, its humanity and inhumanity, its poetry and clichés, its passions and carelessness, is an enfolded and unfolding event, in which there are always slippages from one realm to another (Deleuze, 2000). And there are any number of assemblages that hold individuals the same, that attribute an enduring, unchanging core to them. "Assemblages are living, throbbing confederations that are able to function despite the persistent presence of energies that confound them from within" (Bennett, 2010: 23–24).

New materialism works to make visible/hearable/tangible those movements that hold things the same – inequalities of income and power, for example – as well as the movements that generate creative evolution through openness to the other and the unknown. At the same time as new materialist thought undoes the assumptions of representationalism, it works to find the words and images that evoke the detailed specificity of the more-than-human material world, while acknowledging that things act most powerfully through the senses – the vibrations of colour and touch and smell. The human/more-than-human world constantly changes, unfolding and enfolding, destroying and regenerating itself, as it grieves and endures. As Bennett says, there is always a "swarm of vitalities at play" (2010: 32).

Moving beyond the already known

We are moved when accounts that evoke the detailed specificity of the world transport us elsewhere. In that moment of movement we are lifted out of our lives into that other spacetime. That experience can be euphoric – or very funny, or at the very least, absorbing. Even when we know that the spacetime we are transported to is fictional, we seek it out for the particular pleasure of that movement outside what we think of as ourselves. We go to the movies, on to social media, we read novels, we fall in love – allowing ourselves to be transported elsewhere – an elsewhere that may be more intensely real than the ordinariness and repetitions of our everyday lives. Autopoiesis and sympoiesis – the singular and collective creative acts through which lives are made – and the sympathy on which response-ability depends, require this capacity to move and be moved from one realm to another. Sympathy reaches through intuition towards a reality outside itself.

In 2015 a journalist photographed a dead boy on the beach, and the photo went viral. People living safely on the northern shores of the Mediterranean, and even further north, for whom "refugee" had been an abstract term with no emotional or affective weight, were collectively moved by that photo. They took pity on the plight of the fleeing families in a way they had not done before. The photo transported them to the spacetime of being a dead boy on the beach. There was nothing new in the fact of a drowned boy washed up on the beach; the refugees taking flight across the Mediterranean were extraordinarily vulnerable in their small, leaky boats. But suddenly, there was something in this particular image of a child who had died, that collectively awakened sympathy, and shocked people on the northern shores out of their comfortable ignorance. It was a shock that, in Deleuzian terms, forced them to think. From the point of view of the family, however, it was horrendous that their two-year-old son would be remembered dead rather than alive, and that a film would be made of him dead.

A diffractive methodology that investigated this event would take into account the geopolitical movements that turn people into refugees fleeing their homelands; it would respond to the particular power of the photograph to mobilise change; and it would intra-act with the emotional horror of the boy's family when the photo went viral. The research methodology would itself be movement, and thus part of what it set out to observe and to make sense of. A diffractive analysis might pick up on the tiniest movement, or it may pick up on large sweeps of divergent movements that affect each other. Such research is open to what it doesn't yet know, or even know how to imagine. At the same time, what it comes to know is fragile; it can disappear in the face of other ways of knowing, or in forgetfulness. And it can reappear, always different than it was before.

To pursue the concept of diffraction, Barad "gets *inside* the experiments, unpacking the specific material arrangements to make visible the ever-changing conceptual dimension of matter" (de Freitas, 2017: 741). It is a different getting inside that I will attempt here, an experimental getting inside moments of being and becoming – getting inside their entangled ethico-onto-epistemologies. Such experiments are "risky creative events that reassemble the world" (de Freitas, 2017: 742), that get inside those human and more-than-human lives that are entangled with each other – with bodies such as water, leaky boats, a dead boy.

A diffractive analysis re-situates the specificity of human subjects with-in relations, imbricated in multiple flows and affects. Our utterances about ourselves, including our utterances about our humanity – no matter how fine the autopoiesis or creative details through which we evoke our specificity – are always the products of multiple assemblages. And assemblages are always collective, bringing "into play within us and outside us populations, multiplicities, territories, becomings, affects, events" (Deleuze and Parnet, 1987: 51).

What I hope to make visible here, and usable, is the entangled, always emergent becoming that is *of* the matter and mattering of the world.

Ethics

Ethics is so integral to new materialist thought that Barad coined the term ethico-onto-epistemology in order to make clear that a new materialist researcher is never free of responsibility. Research encounters dislodged from habituated thoughts and practices are no random matter, though they may be unpredictable. The concept of entanglement brings with it an entirely different conception of ethics. In place of the institutional ethics that tie down the research event to controlled and predictable practices and outcomes, new materialist ethics, in its unpredictability, never lets the researcher off the hook of considering how their emergent thoughts and actions matter.

In place of researchers who stand back from the material that is being researched, assessing it and judging it from a distant vantage point, new materialist researchers are not separate or separable from the field of study, in which they mobilise all their senses, touching and being open to being touched by the human and more-than-human world that they research and write about. With-in a quantum relationality,

> Touch becomes the fundamental relation of the world – a quivering quantum tug that holds us together, rather than a classical physical collision encounter. [Barad] claims that this quantum touch stretches across the inhuman field of virtual indeterminacy and can furnish an ethics adequate to the world.
>
> (de Freitas, 2017: 747)

This book is in pursuit of such an ethics.

I end this first chapter with an encounter written in the form of a poem:

Cutting loose
I rested safe in
who I was to you
          what it was possible
to be was
in your voice   your skin
          your eyes

I knew that when
I died   the words
that would tell
who I had been
would come from your mouth

  and my sons might know
me then   through
your eyes   and the particular
quality of your care

then you grew tired of me
    bored   the idea of
seeing me palled
    there was nothing in
my eyes   my skin
my mouth   you wanted

I was dead already

      there was nothing to say...

the memories of conjoint longings
    stories told
of suffering

intermittent   flowings forth   into
the molecular detail of each other's
    lives
were mine alone to keep

          or to finally set adrift on the tide

I wonder, now, why that friendship, in particular, was so hard to let go of. Why had I come to believe that this friend, above all others, knew me as others did not, or could not? In a Cartesian version of what it is to be human, we can only ever know ourselves, and cannot know what lies outside ourselves – so "the other" must always remain opaque to us. But we are also opaque to ourselves. It is, at least in part, in the gaze of the other, in their listening and responding that we come to life.

The friend to whom the poem was addressed was a photographer. Her photos of me were a gift to me of myself. They meant that I could see what she saw. But more than that, I had become whatever it was that the photos had captured *in my responding to her.* I was not alone in this. All her photographic subjects displayed a particular life-fullness in responding to her. It was that subject who had responded to her that I wanted to continue to be.

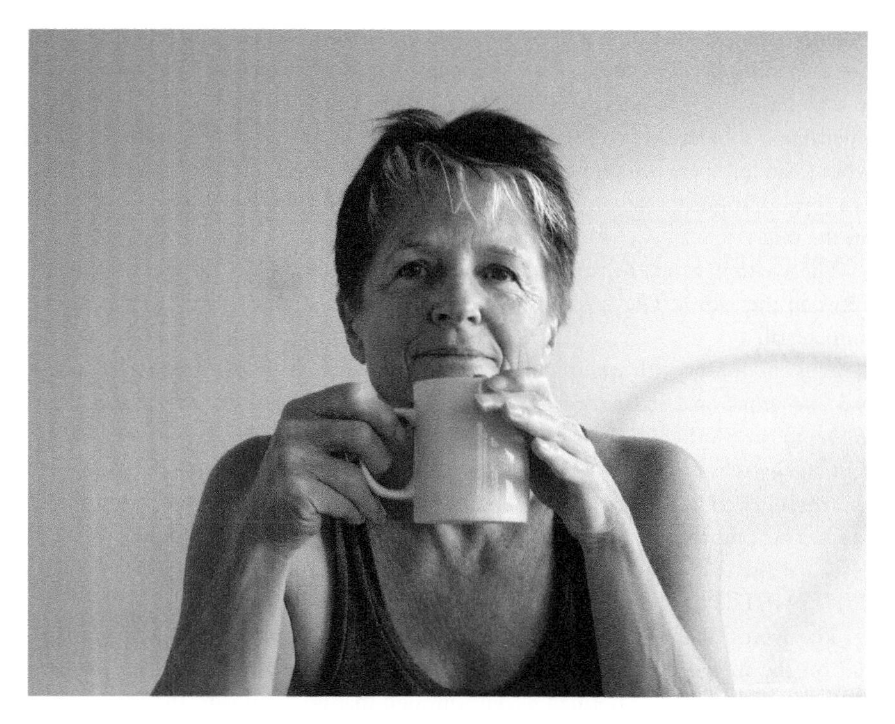

FIGURE 1.1 The gift. Portrait of the author.
Photographer anon., 2006.

The more formal photos that she gave me in printed form lie in an envelope in a deep drawer containing hundreds of photos. The less formal photos, like this one, that she gave me, are digital copies, and they sit on my desktop and are the only photos I keep of myself. They have what Bennett calls thing-power: "the curious ability of inanimate things to animate, to act, to produce effects dramatic and subtle" (Bennett, 2010: 6).

Each photo holds one moment of the changing, infinite alterity of that self. In the capture of that moment of relational flow, this photo creates the illusion that this is who I "really am". And yes, I really was this, in response to someone who gazed at her subjects in a loving way. I loved that loving gaze, and I loved what I could become in response. Looking at the photo of myself is what Barad calls self-touching.

> *self-touching is an encounter with the infinite alterity of the self. Matter is an enfolding, an involution, it cannot help touching itself, and in this self-touching it comes in contact with the infinite alterity that it is* ... What is being called into question here is the very nature of the "self," and in terms of not just being but also time. That is, in an important sense, the self is dispersed/diffracted through time and being.
>
> (Barad, 2015: 158–159)

And precisely because of that dispersion and diffraction, and the scattering of alterities through space and time, it was this one particular alterity that she offered me, in which my body responded to that loving gaze, that I wanted to hold. But when I became a subject she no longer desired as a friend or as a photographic subject, what I had left were the photos and an unbearable sense of loss. I turned to writing as a form of inquiry that would enable a transformation, a willing dispersal of "self" on the tide.

The written words became agents in the encounter, as did the physical spaces between the words. The spaces provided a pause, a breath, a break; they were not immaterial.

This encounter with writing materially enveloped me and made possible a physical and emotional letting go: "language is a kind of haptic/touch relation that *inheres* in the world and perhaps *expresses* the world" (de Freitas, 2017: 744). We are touched by words just as we are touched by human and more-than-human others. We are touched by events, and by the (in)animate. "Touch in a postquantum world reaches beyond the conventional phenomenological framing of hapticity and suggests a massive intimacy across a spectrum of possible envelopments" (de Freitas, 2017: 744). The poet does not stand alone, and nor does the poem.

The words of the final line of my poem, when I found them, drawing as they did on the image of the tide, had, for me, in that moment, an affective power I couldn't have named or defined except through that poetic image; the force of the image seemed miraculous; my body released its desire to be known by this friend; as I wrote them I watched with amazement as the sense of loss washed out on that imagined tide.

There is no formula I know of that might tell how such words might be found. For me it was trial and error and an intense desire to remove myself from the state of loss that had taken me over. I wanted to transport myself, in effect, out of the space–time of abandonment and loss. It might seem ironic, and inconsistent for someone who has been exploring poststructuralist theory and now new materialism, to have been so attached to being known – being recognised. It's interesting to think about the way in which, time and again, we hand to our loved ones the power to secure the elusive, slippery, multiplicity that is known as "oneself". Perhaps it is that very slipperiness and multiplicity that makes us yearn for being recognised as someone in particular, someone who is worthy of love – of the relationality we depend on: "desire cannot be eliminated from the core of being – it is threaded through it" (Barad, 2015: 160).

The poem is an experiment in living as- and writing-as-inquiry, in which I turned to the poetics of writing to create movement out of the space–time I had been thrust into. It is onto-epistemological in so far as the words and the bodies, human bodies and more-than-human bodies – the ocean tide, the photos, the bodies that love and are lost, are not separate from each other; it offers a way of thinking and doing the grief of ending a friendship. It stays with the moment. It endures. In doing so it highlights the dependencies that friendship generates, at the same time as it takes the writer/reader materially into the experience of that dependency, and then into the ethico-onto-epistemology of letting the dependency go. The material world here is made up of two women's bodies, the materiality of the poem itself, the photo and the tide. Its ethics lie in the Deleuzian question: What is it to be this? What is the peculiar nature of the dependency and the letting go of that dependency? Deleuze advocates a non-judgemental openness to oneself and the other; he is interested in generating movement beyond fixed places, through finding ways to think the unthinkable. While warning against "wildly destratifying" (Deleuze and Guattari, 1987: 160), he is interested in an ethics that can unlock fixed lines of descent and give rise to differenciation – to becoming different from what one was before (Deleuze, 1980).

In each of the chapters that follow, I pick up and elaborate on the concepts and ideas I have explored in Chapter 1: vital materiality, the conditions of creative production, thing-power, diffractive methodology, refrains, recognition, sympathy, intuition and the flow in-between, ethico-onto-epistemology and the creative invention of new possibilities.

References

Barad, K. 2003. Posthumanist performativity: How matter comes to matter. *Signs: Journal of Women in Culture and Society*, 28(3), 801–831.

Barad, K. 2008. Queer causation and the ethics of mattering. In M. J. Hyrd and N. Giffney (eds), *Queering the Non/Human*. Taylor & Francis Group. ProQuest Ebook, 247–352.

Barad, K. 2015. On touching the inhuman that therefore I am (v1.1). In K. Stakemeier and S. Witzgall (eds), *Power of Material/Politics of Materiality*. Zurich, SW: Diaphanes, 153–164.

Bennett, J. 2010. *Vibrant Matter. A Political Ecology of Things*. Durham, NC: Duke University Press.

Bergson, H. 1998. *Creative Evolution* (trans. A. Mitchell). Mineola, NY: Dover Publications Inc.

Bright, D. 2018. Signs to be developed: experiments in writing. In S. Riddle, D. Bright and E. Honan (eds), *Writing with Deleuze in the Academy: Creating Monsters*. Singapore: Springer, 95–105.

Davies, B. and Gannon, S. (eds) 2006. *Doing Collective Biography*. Maidenhead, UK: Open University Press.

de Freitas, E. 2017. Karen Barad's quantum ontology and posthuman ethics. Rethinking the concept of relationality. *Qualitative Inquiry*, 23(9), 741–748.

Deleuze, G. 1980. *Cours Vincennes, 12/21/1980*, http://www.webdeleuze.com/php/texte.php?cle=190andgroupe=Spinoza andlangue=2) (accessed 10 February 2010).

Deleuze, G. 2000. *Proust and Signs* (trans. R. Howard). Minneapolis, MN: University of Minnesota Press.

Deleuze, G. and Guattari, F. 1987. *A Thousand Plateaus. Capitalism and Schizophrenia* (trans. B. Massumi). Minneapolis, MN: University of Minnesota Press.

Deleuze, G. and Parnet, C.. 1987. *Dialogues 11*, Revised Edition, (trans. H. Tomlinson and B. Habberjam). New York: Columbia University Press.

Doerr, A. 2005. *About Grace*. London: Fourth Estate.

Grosz, E. 2011. *Becoming Undone: Darwinian Reflections on Life, Politics, and Art*. Durham NC: Duke University Press.

Haraway, D. 1997. *Modest_Witness@Second_Millennium: Female_Man©_Meets_Oncomouse™* (2nd edn 2018). New York and London: Routledge.

Massumi, B. 2015. The supernormal animal. In R. Grusin (ed.), *The Nonhuman Turn*. Minneapolis, MN: University of Minnesota Press, 1–17.

Riddle, S., Bright, D. and Honan, E. (eds), 2018. *Writing with Deleuze in the Academy: Creating Monsters*. Singapore: Springer.

St Pierre, E. 2019. Post qualitative inquiry in an ontology of immanence. *Qualitative Inquiry*, 25(1), 3–16.

Vannini, P. 2015. Non-representational ethnography: New ways of animating lifeworlds. *Cultural Geographies*, 22(2), 317–327.

Wyatt, J. 2019. *Therapy, Stand-up, and the Gesture of Writing*. New York: Routledge.

Wyatt, J., Gale, K., Gannon, S. & Davies, B. 2011. *Deleuze and Collaborative Writing: An Immanent Plane of Composition*. New York: Peter Lang.

2

VITAL MATERIALITY

> In which I explore the intra-active mattering of humans and more-than-humans, drawing primarily on the work of Barad and Bennett and also Deleuze and Guattari. I ponder how we might generate ethical encounters that are open and alive to the vital materiality of more-than-human others. I propose an ethics based on response-ability and on an understanding of our mutual engagement, our affective co-existence, with the more-than-human world. I interrupt the striations of unquestioned human dominance and exploitation of more-than-human others, and explore, in place of those striations, a sensuous enchantment with the material world.

In the first chapter I opened up the practices of auto- and sympoiesis – the creative acts through which lives are made. And I discussed the sympathy on which response-ability depends, and which requires the capacity to move, and be moved, from one realm to another. I also explored the power of images when they are put to work in the analysis of a diffractive encounter, in a poetic experiment in living, and in moving from stuck places. I began the work of unpicking the way we routinely mobilise Enlightenment thought to separate out and individualise human subjects as if they were entities that exist entirely inside their own finite borders, and I worked with the concept of becoming, in which life is intra-active and emergent.

I will ponder, in this chapter, the *matter and mattering* of an encounter between an adult, a child and a pond. The *matter* of my three participants, in this analysis, is not a fixed substance; rather, in Barad's definition, "*matter is substance in its intra-active becoming – not a thing, but a doing, a congealing of agency. Matter is a stabilizing and destabilizing process of iterative intra-activity*" (2003: 822). Barad further defines *intra-activity* as "relationships between multiple bodies (both human and non-human) that are understood not to have clear or distinct boundaries from one another: rather, they are always affecting or being affected by each other in an interdependent and mutual relationship" (Barad, 2007: 152).

Encounters, in a new materialist analysis, are no longer a matter of active, agentic humans acting on a material world that has no agency; each participant has agency; each affects the other; and each depends on the other. The matter and mattering of encounters, in this conceptualisation, involve multiple relationships among humans, animals and earth others, where the boundaries between them are permeable and in flux. The automatic dominance of one group over another, or of one individual over another, and the automatic assumption of human dominance over the other-than-human world, are called radically into question. Even dominance over oneself and one's own matter, of mind over body, demands further thought.

This opens up the possibility of a major shift in thinking about adult–child relations. Adult domination is integral to the usual modes of interaction between adults and children, where adults are likely to approach children with the intent of managing and mastering them, and children's activity is often construed as learning mastery over their own bodies and over their emotions. That mastering and dominating is based on a morality that determines what we *should* each become; it's a morality that imposes "from a superior vantage point a definition of Being that presumes to judge and find lacking" (Wyatt and Davies, 2011: 107). Ethics framed in terms of such moral judgements, will most likely be focused on curbing adult violence, and maximising children's development of mastery over themselves, and over objects. A new materialist ethics, in contrast, is interested in the opening up of creativity, and in fostering engagement with the not-yet-known. It is interested in the processes of intra-active becomings, and in our responsibility and response-ability in those mutual engagements. What we do matters, how we respond matters; we are not *in* the world but *of* the world, and our intra-actions are integral to the always emergent making of the world.

This shift away from human separation and domination, towards an emergent, interdependent liveliness, is ontological (we no longer have discrete bodies), epistemological (we have new concepts to think with), and it is ethical (where ethical action can no longer be accomplished by following the rules of a particular moral order, but must be accomplished again and again as we respond to each other).

People and things

In reconceptualising things as having vitality, in Bennett's terms, and agency, in Barad's terms, the human subject is also re-conceptualised in its liveliness, in its capacity to respond to the liveliness of the world, and in its belonging to that world. Barad advocates "the ongoing practice of being open and alive to each meeting, each intra-action, so that we might use our ability to respond, our responsibility, to help awaken, to breathe life into ever new possibilities for living justly" (Barad, 2007: x). In those intra-actions we do not remain ontologically or epistemologically separate from those we are alive to; we cannot remain unaffected; we cannot remain what we were before, or remain tied, to whatever extent we were so, to particular categories and associated identities.

Things, in Bennett's analysis, are what we encounter when we give up our epistemological domination of objects, when we stop trying to make them fit into our preconceived notions of what they are, and come to experience them as uncanny (Bennett, 2010: 2). In such an encounter, human subjects recognise the inappropriateness of, and the negation involved in, objectifying the other. They search instead for ways of knowing things – of knowing the power of things to affect and to be affected – a form of knowing that enables them to greet that which is rising up toward them (Cixous, 1976; Mitchell, 2005; Thomson and Davies, 2019).

This chapter is an exploration of that intra-active practice of being open and alive to the uncanny, and what it is in the world that rises up to meet us, inviting a response from us, and expanding us as it does so. It is about being open to the possibility of softening one's borders – or, rather, becoming aware of the ways in which those borders are already more soft, more permeable, than we might have thought – as are the borders of the things – the material vitalities – around us. The matter of ourselves, then, and the matter of those others, human and more-than-human, "*is substance in its intra-active becoming*" (Barad, 2003: 822).

The story I begin with is of a boy, his mother, a pond, and the intra-actions between them. I was sitting by one of the ponds in the Botanic Garden, near my home in Sydney, when this small drama began to unfold.

A small boy picked up a large palm frond, much bigger than himself, and threw it into the pond. Just before he threw it, his mother, sitting nearby, yelled "No!" He then picked up a very large stick and glanced at her. She shouted "No!" again, and he threw it into the pond. The third time, he picked up a smaller stick, and when his mother yelled "No!" he hid it surreptitiously behind his back, glancing at me, as if to say, "See how cunning I am, she doesn't know I am still holding it." The mother turned her face away from the boy and the pond; her body registered futility and exhaustion. The boy threw his smaller stick and then began looking for a larger one. He continued to throw sticks while his mother looked away, but his game seemed to be less fun, once the edge of danger, which her shouts had given to his game, had ceased.

Quite apart from the fact that my own peace by the pond was shattered, I was distressed at the harm that the boy's game was doing to the pond and to its inhabitants. I doubted that the pond was able to accommodate the boy's careless play. Those huge, stringy palm fronds take many years to decompose, and the pond, unlike the ocean, has no means of ejecting them. He was treating the pond as if it had no life of its own, and no capacity to suffer, and as if it had nothing to offer him other than as a passive receptacle designed for his pleasure.

The habit of throwing waste matter into the waterways is a centuries old practice. The history of human domination over this particular waterway is at least 230 years old. The freshwater spring in Sydney Harbour made it an ideal place for the First Fleeters, in 1788, to set up the British Colony of New South Wales. My ancestor,

David Collins, was among those First Fleeters; he was Judge Advocate and Secretary to the Governor. He wrote in his journal about his encounter with this same place:

> The spot chosen for this encampment was at the head of the cove, near the run of fresh water, which stole silently through a very thick wood, the stillness of which had then, for the first time since the creation, been interrupted by the rude sound of the labourer's axe, and the downfall of its ancient inhabitants; a stillness and tranquillity which from that day were to give place to the voice of labour, the confusion of camps and towns, and the "busy hum of its new possessors".
>
> (Collins, 1798: 4)

My ancestor's account of the first fleeters' encounter with this place, and the boy's encounter with the pond have a characteristic in common – an apparent profound lack of sympathy for their more-than-human others.

Having cleared the forest, the colonists set up their houses along the stream, then threw all their rubbish and excreta into it, polluting it so thoroughly that eventually they had to abandon it, and seek an alternative water supply.

David Collins was eager to be recognized by his British masters as a worthy subject. In responding to published eulogies offered to British soldiers, victorious in battle in other parts of the Empire, David Collins asked why he and his fellow officers, who were building the colony of New South Wales, might not also be recognized as British subjects who were contributing to the glory of Empire. Surely, he argued in his journal, bringing British civilization to a savage world, and transforming the convicted British outcasts into decent men and women, was a glorious enterprise?

> though labouring at a distance, and in an humbler scene, yet the good, the glory, and the aggrandizement of our country were prime considerations with us. And why should the colonists of New South Wales be denied the merit of endeavouring to promote [British values], by establishing civilization in the savage world; by animating the children of idleness and vice to habits of laborious and honest industry; and by shewing the world that to Englishmen no difficulties are insuperable?
>
> (Collins, 1798: 55)

The boy, too, I suspect, was eager for recognition – from his mother, or even from a stranger.

It is all too easy to stand in judgement of the colonists, and of the boy, and to find them wanting, in not living up to ideals I might measure them against. But moral judgement of my ancestor, or of the boy, or of the exhausted mother, is not relevant here. Moral judgement would serve as a self-protective measure, placing a barrier between me, as the one who judges, and my ancestor and the boy, who are judged. Moral judgement abjects the other, spitting them out as if they are not part of oneself, "(which is never one or self)" (Barad, 2014: 182). If I engaged in such judgement, as I confess I did for some minutes after I witnessed the boy-stick-mother-pond assemblage, I would effectively reinforce my self-righteous borders, shutting myself off from the entangled intra-actions of the assemblage and from any understanding of colonisation, or of the boy's encounter with the pond.

Deleuze suggests that, rather than moral judgement, we ask of the other "What is it to be this? What makes the just-thisness of you, in this moment?"

> You ask yourself how is that possible? How is this possible in an internal way? In other words, you relate the thing or the statement to the mode of existence that it implies, that it envelops in itself. How must it be in order to say that? What manner of Being does this imply? You seek the enveloped modes of existence, and not the transcendent values.
>
> (Deleuze, 1980: np)

To ask that question, how is it possible, in an internal way, I want to go back in time a little, to a day by the pond before the boy-stick-mother assemblage formed itself. I want to bring the thing-power, or congealed agency, of the pond more clearly into my story, as another *actant* in the assemblage. An actant, or source of action, "can be human or not, or most likely, a combination of both" (Bennett, 2010: 9): "an actant never really acts alone. Its efficacy or agency always depends on the collaboration, cooperation, or interactive interference of many bodies and forces" (Bennett, 2010: 21).

The concept Bennett works with, similar to Barad's intra-action, is "shared, vital materiality" (Bennett, 2010: 14), which can open up among humans, and among human and more-than-human others. These concepts put the violent hierarchy of anthropocentrism and essentialised human subjectivities under erasure. Bennett asks, "Why advocate the vitality of matter?" and she answers:

> Because my hunch is that the image of dead or thoroughly instrumentalized matter feeds human hubris … by preventing us from detecting (seeing, hearing, smelling, tasting, feeling) a fuller range of nonhuman powers circulating around and within human bodies.
>
> (Bennett, 2010: ix)

And so, I turn to my own story of intra-action, of shared vital materiality, with the pond, a vital materiality that was disrupted with the boy-stick-mother-pond event.

I am lying on the bench beside the pond. The pond has lavender-coloured water lilies, a family of dusky moorhens and two brown ducks. There are ibis, too, who fly in to enjoy the shade at the edge of the pond, sheltered as it is by an overhanging giant water gum and a vast weeping lilly pilly. The ibis migrated to the city decades ago when there was a severe inland drought and, like me, they never went back. Nearby there is a coffee shop and there are chairs and tables outside.

Lying on my bench, looking up through the canopy of leaves, I am enveloped and restored by the pond. Its uncanny energy is not something I can represent in words.

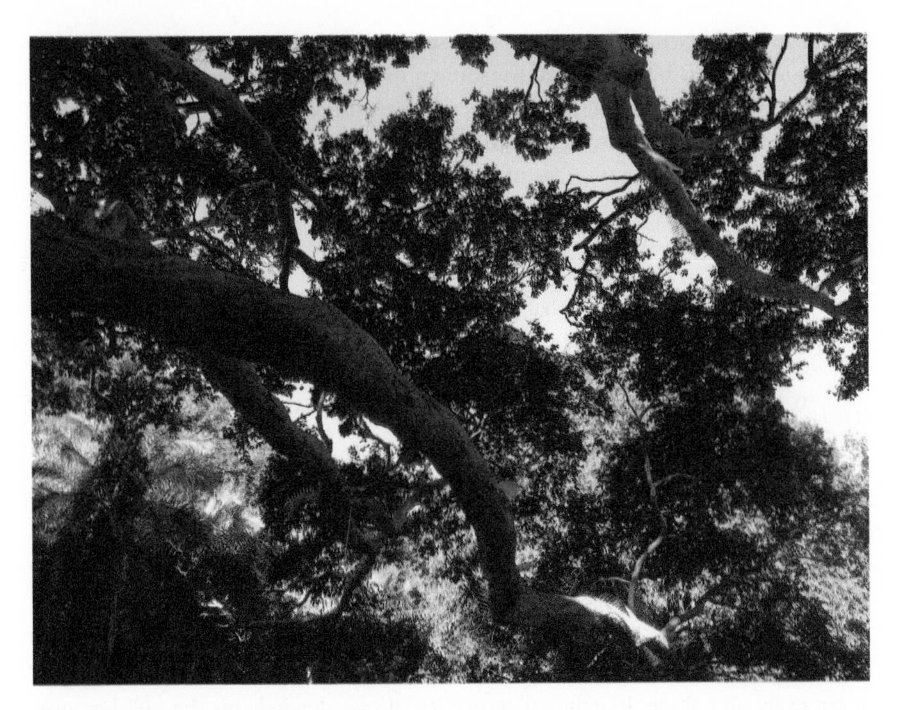

FIGURE 2.1 The Giant Water Gum canopy.
The Royal Botanic Garden, Sydney. Photograph by Bronwyn Davies, 2018.

The pond is alive with its own life, its own means of staying alive and supporting the life of the birds, and the life of the trees. I feel its life-sustaining energy lapping out and enveloping me. I become, for the time I lie there on the bench, a member of the pond, included in its life. The affect flows between one body and another – back and forth between me and the pond – an uncanny exchange, so subtle that it lies before awareness, and resists representation even while it draws me in to become part of it, penetrating my borders.

It is difficult to find words for the thing-power or vital materiality of the pond. I have no doubt that the matter of my body was affected by the pond, but I don't have the concepts to adequately "acknowledge the obscure but ubiquitous intensity of [its] impersonal affect" (Bennett, 2010: xiii). It is through the work of artists and writers who use syntax, lines and colours to "raise lived perceptions to percepts and lived affections to affect" (Deleuze and Guattari, 1994: 170) that the intra-action might find expression, making legible the intensities and flows in between the materiality of my body and the vital materiality of the pond.

Deleuze and Guattari (1994: 170) contemplate the writerly and artistic process of raising "lived perceptions to percepts and lived affections to affect". Of the work of novelists, they write, for example:

> The novel has often risen to the percept – not perception of the moor in Hardy but the moor as percept; oceanic percepts in Melville; urban percepts,

> or those of the mirror, in Virginia Woolf. The landscape sees ... Characters can only exist, and the author can only create them, because they do not perceive but have passed into the landscape and are themselves part of the compound of sensations. Ahab really does have perceptions of the sea, but only because he has entered into a relationship with Moby Dick that makes him becomingwhale and forms a compound of sensations that no longer needs anyone: ocean. It is Mrs. Dalloway who perceives the town – but because she has passed into the town like "a knife through everything" and becomes imperceptible herself.
>
> (Deleuze and Guattari, 1994: 168–169)

Such novelists, working with affects and percepts, generate individuals and landscapes that are co-implicated, as mutually entangled agencies, human subjects becoming ocean, or moor or city – or in my case, becoming pond (Davies and Gannon, 2013).

I call on my writerly skill, then, to move from affection and perception to percept and affect, with some help from the photographic images of multiple moments in which I have become pond.

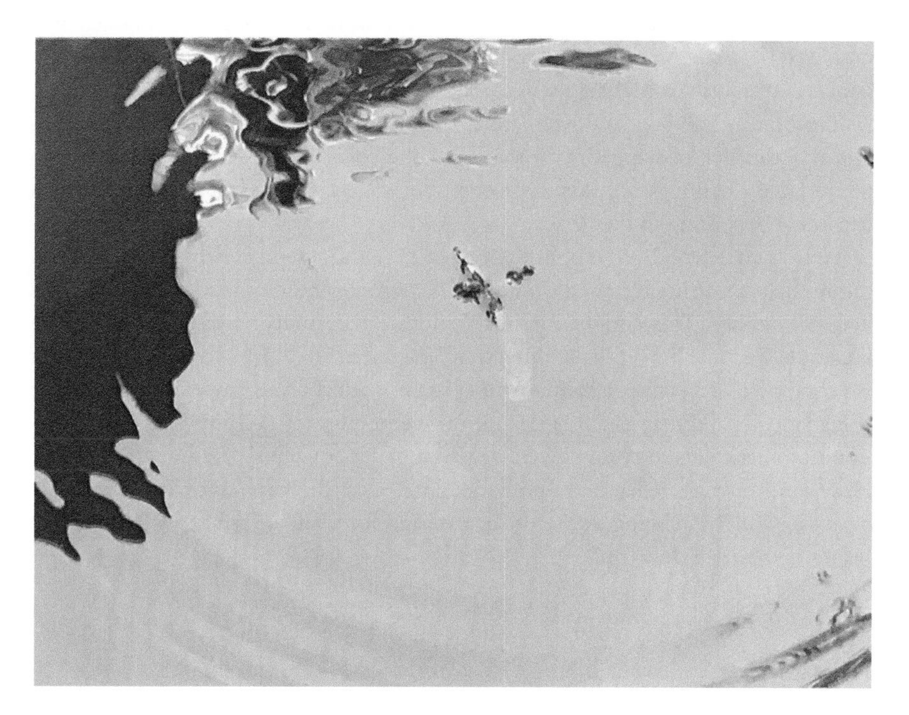

FIGURE 2.2 Dragonfly on the surface of the pond.
The Royal Botanic Garden, Sydney. Photograph by Bronwyn Davies, 2020.

At first as I lay on the bench, looking up through the canopy, I had wondered how I could make sense of the agency of the pond. What was it doing? How did it affect me? Was it aware of me? I gazed at the surface of the pond, at the play of light on its surface, I photographed it, I listened to it, I waited. In Nancy's (2007) terms, I stretched my ears and all my senses. I was affected by it, without being able to say how – how it was that my body felt restored, enfolded. My eyes and ears and skin had opened themselves to its vital materiality. I came to know the pond, and myself, as neither one nor self – without borders, without ascendance, without mastery, and without words. I began to know what the pond could do by entering into composition with it. As Deleuze and Guattari say: "We know nothing about a body until we know what it can do, in other words, what its affects are, how they can or cannot enter into composition with other affects, with the affects of another body" (Deleuze and Guattari, 1987: 257). In this reconfigured assemblage of shared materiality with the pond, what comes to matter?

Barad (2007: 396) argues that "[i]ntra-acting responsibly as part of the world means taking account of the entangled phenomena that are intrinsic to the world's vitality, and being responsive to the possibilities that might help us and it flourish". In becoming aware of my shared vibrant materiality with the pond, I came to understand quite differently how the life of the pond matters. Together, we became part of the "entangled phenomena that are intrinsic to the world's vitality" (Barad, 2007: 396). I was not separate from the pond, but "*of* the world in its ongoing intra-activity" (Barad, 2003: 828). As such, my responsibility toward the pond became more than a bunch of idealistic words, but a will to care for the pond as being *of* me, and me *of* it.

The boy and his stick and palm-frond throwing had not just shattered my peacefulness – the lack of sympathy for the pond, the consequent inability to respond to the pond as anything more than a receptacle, was a lack of sympathy for my own expanded becoming in that space.

How then, I wondered, might the boy-stick-pond assemblage have shifted from the re-citation of mastery and dominance to one of inter-dependence and shared material vitality? How might the boy "cultivate the ability to discern nonhuman vitality, to become perceptually open to it" (Bennett, 2010: 14)? In trying to answer that question I run again into my own epistemological limits; my existing language is inadequate, and may even work against me, because of the way "conceptualization automatically obscures the inadequacy of its concepts" (Bennett, 2010: 14). How can I envisage what an ethical encounter with the stick-throwing boy might become, while remaining aware of the limiting force of the concepts I, or he and his mother, might draw on?

Cultivating sympathy

In Chapter 1, I defined sympathy as reaching through intuition to a reality outside itself. Sympathy depends on *emergent listening*, a listening that is open to realities that are not yet known (Davies, 2014). Listening-as-usual, in contrast, picks up on, and lodges itself within, the striations that make up the orderly, everyday world. Listening-as-usual to the boy/mother encounter is to hear, for example, a wilfully naughty boy and a negligent mother, and to conclude that the boy needs to be taught to obey his mother and the mother needs to acquire some parenting skills. Both mother and boy can be exposed to moral judgement and found to fall short. Listening-as-usual might also produce a hearing of the pond as an object of no consequence, as no more than a receptacle for waste matter, or alternatively, as having magical-natural powers which it can draw on to process the rubbish. None of these would save the pond from being abjected.

Listening-as-usual can ask questions only in the terms of already laid down concepts, and in mobilising them, cement both the concepts' certainties and limitations. To interrupt those certainties and limitations, Bennett suggests "What is also needed is a cultivated, patient, sensory attentiveness to nonhuman forces operating outside and inside the human body" (Bennett, 2010: xiv).

Emergent listening is open to what it doesn't know; its borders are open. In some senses it works against the self of the listener and the desire for fixed, striated, already-given concepts and methods. Through emergent listening, we open ourselves to entangled vital materialities, our own and others', and to an awareness of their capacity to affect each other: "Our capacity to affect each other, to enter into composition with others both enhances our specificity and expands our capacity for thought and action" (Davies, 2014: 20). Agency in such an encounter is distributed and multiple, and within that entangled multiplicity, each participant is emergent and vividly alive – open to being affected, not just by words, or within the terms of existing relations, but by percepts and affects, by things in the world (both human and more-than-human), whose force may be both uncanny and vital.

Living on and near the pond is a family of moorhens with their red legs and faces, and two ducks diving, tails in the air, foraging for food at the bottom of the pond. The reflections on the surface of the pond are exquisite and endlessly in motion, ruffled by the ducks, moorhens and ibis, and ruffled by breezes and the passage of water over the small waterfalls. It reflects the surrounding trees, the sky and clouds.

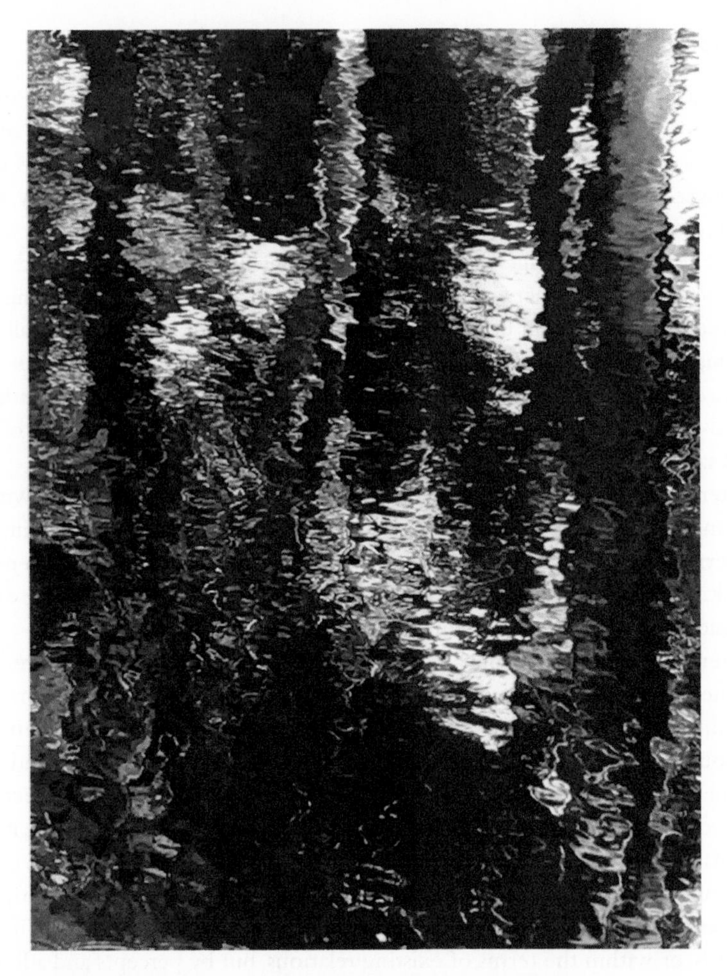

FIGURE 2.3 Uncanny vitality: ripples on the surface of the pond. The Royal Botanic Garden, Sydney. Photograph by Bronwyn Davies, 2020.

Attending to the pond, entering into composition with it, the mother's vitality might have revived, and perhaps her son would have joined her in the task of opening up a quite different assemblage, one that was open to the unexpected, and the uncanny – to the vital materiality of the pond.

There is a gently trickling waterfall that takes water out of the pond, around which the ducks, moorhens and ibis gather. The ibis's feet, as it stands on the railing, has toes that curl first around the rail like fingers and thumb, then when it turns it shifts all toes, like our toes, in the same direction. Mother and son might have marvelled together at the fact that the ibis's feet, while made up of the same bones as his own feet, have got the dexterity of a hand as well as the strength of a foot.

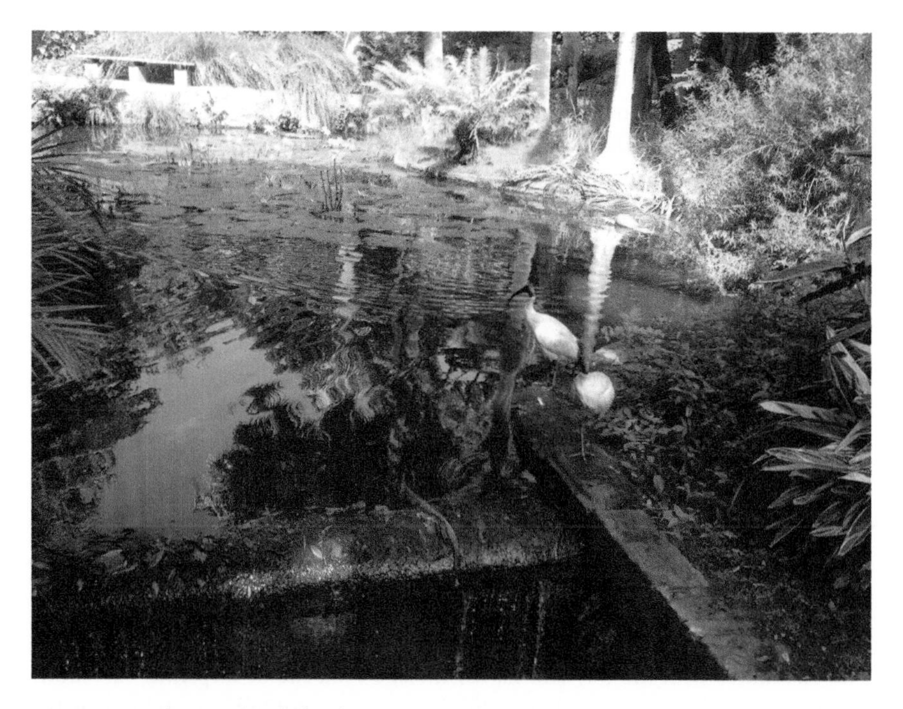

FIGURE 2.4 The pond and the ibis.
The Royal Botanic Garden, Sydney. Photograph by Bronwyn Davies, 2018.

To wonder and to listen to the pond with all one's senses is to allow the pond into oneself through ears and eyes and skin. In opening myself to the kind of wondering that might have enticed the boy to stretch his eyes and ears and skin, I ask where does the water come from into the pond? I discover a series of waterfalls and bridges, and still further up, I find the pipes through which the water flows in, from under the city. I wonder where the water comes from before that? Does it come from the same water-source as the Tank Stream that the First Fleeters found in 1788? Did the building of the city and the sealing of the roads destroy the wetlands that supplied the water in the first place? Does Sydney have any wetlands left? Can I discover more about wetlands and the work they do in filtering the water? Can I learn more about the way sandstone acts as a water filter? Were any of the sandstone walls, still here, built by the convicts who came out on the First Fleet? Who were those convicts and how did their lives matter? Some of those questions I pursued in *New Lives in an Old Land* (2019).

Listening and wondering can work to interrupt the striations of unquestioned human dominance and exploitation. But stretching the senses needs more than fact-finding to move from perceptions to percepts and affections to affects. To open oneself to the more-than-human other needs more than wondering; it requires an openness to the possibility of auto- and sympoietic, sensuous enchantments.

Such an openness enables the letting go of the desire for "identity" (of one and self) and opens instead the possibility of experiencing oneself as a vital materiality, and as such, one of many things in intra-action with a world of things: "human power is itself a kind of thing-power ... [Our bodily materiality can be understood as] lively and self-organizing, rather than as passive or mechanical means under the direction of something nonmaterial, that is, an active soul or mind" (Bennett, 2010: 10).

I began this chapter with a chance encounter by a pond, open to the pond, but at first not open to the boy-mother-pond assemblage on that particular day. I was peculiarly affected by the boy and his participation in the abjection of the waterway. As Schulte observes of such chance encounters and their relevance to our research:

> we don't always have the power to decide which problems receive our attention, nor do we have the leverage to decide how long we linger with them. Rather, problems arise from and are contingent [on] the encounters we have with something or someone, encounters that force thought to rise up and that move us to think something we never thought we could ever think.
>
> (Schulte, 2016: 147)

The encounter with the boy and his assemblage took me in surprising directions, toward new ways of thinking about ethical encounters, not just among humans, but also with the more-than-human. The trail of thought and affect brought me to a point similar to Guattari when he said that the problems of ecology are "as much a matter of culture-and-psyche formation as ... of watershed management and air quality protection" (cited in Bennett, 2010: 114). I came to an understanding that our capacity for ethical encounters with others, both human and more-than-human, depends on some of those shifts in understanding that come from a co-mingling and entering into a shared composition with more-than-human, animal and earth others. Bennett offers a challenge to old refrains that emerge from this new-found appreciation of matter:

> Each human is a heterogeneous compound of wonderfully vibrant, dangerously vibrant, matter. If matter itself is lively, then not only is the difference between subjects and objects minimized, but the status of the shared materiality of all things is elevated ... Such newfound attentiveness to matter and its powers will not solve the problem of human exploitation or oppression, but it can inspire a greater sense of the extent to which all bodies are kin in the sense of inextricably enmeshed in a dense network of relations.
>
> (Bennett, 2010: 12–13)

And so... I have invited you here, to sit by the pond with me and to co-mingle with it, and with the ibis, the trees, a mother and a boy. I have asked you to come with me in imagining a world not full of moral judgement and lack, but one full of wonder and response-ability. I have asked you to shed some old refrains and open yourself up to new ways of imagining your place in the world, and new ways of listening to the world – and to wondering what is possible.

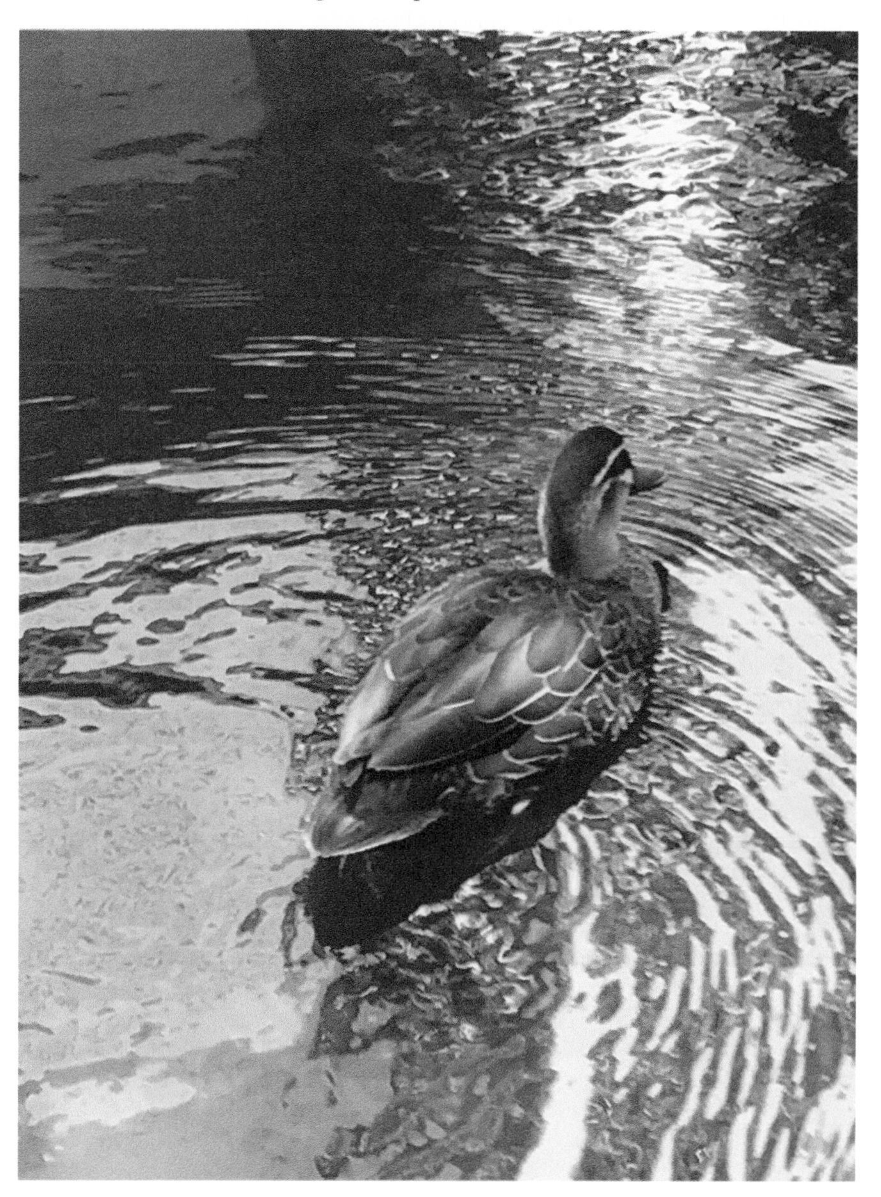

FIGURE 2.5 The duck and the pond.
The Royal Botanic Garden, Sydney. Photograph by Bronwyn Davies, 2020.

References

Barad, K. 2003. Posthumanist performativity: Toward an understanding of how matter comes to matter. *Signs: Journal of Women in Culture and Society*, 28(3), 801–831.

Barad, K. 2007. *Meeting the Universe Halfway: Quantum Physics and the Entanglement of Matter and Meaning*. Durham, NC: Duke University Press.

Barad, K. 2014. Diffracting diffraction: cutting together-apart, *Parallax*, 20(3), 168–187.

Bennett, J. 2010. *Vibrant Matter. A Political Ecology of Things*. Durham, NC: Duke University Press.

Cixous, H. 1976. Fiction and its phantoms: A reading of Freud's *Das Unheimliche* (The "Uncanny"), (trans. R. Denommé), *New Literary History*, 7(3), 525–548.

Collins, D. 1798. *An Account of the English Colony in New South Wales*. Vol. 1. Sydney: A.H. and A.W. Reed.

Davies, B. 2014. *Listening to Children: Being and Becoming*. London: Routledge.

Davies, B. 2019. *New Lives in an Old Land. Re-turning to the Colonization of New South Wales through Stories of my Parents and their Ancestors*. Sydney, NSW: Ornythorhynchus Paradoxus Books.

Davies, B. 2020. Pondering the pond: Ethical encounters with children. In C. Schulte (ed.), *Ethics and Research with Young Children: New Perspectives*. London: Bloomsbury Academic, 147–161.

Davies, B. and Gannon, S. 2013. Collective biography and the entangled enlivening of being, *International Review of Qualitative Research*, 5(4), 357–376.

Deleuze, G. 1980. *Cours Vincennes*, 21 December 1980. http://www.webdeleuze.com/php/texte.php?cle=190andgroupe=Spinozaandlangue=2 (accessed 10 February 2010)

Deleuze, G. and Guattari, F. 1987. *A Thousand Plateaus: Capitalism and Schizophrenia*, (trans. B. Massumi). London: Athlone Press.

Deleuze, G. and Guattari, F. 1994. *What Is Philosophy?* (trans. H. Tomlinson and G. Burchell). New York: Columbia University Press.

Mitchell, W. J. T. 2005. *What Do Pictures Want? The Lives and Loves of Images*. Chicago, IL: Chicago University Press.

Nancy, J.-L. 2007. *Listening* (trans. C. Mandell). New York: Fordham University Press.

Schulte, C. M. 2016. Possible worlds: Deleuzian ontology and the project of listening in children's drawing. *Cultural Studies <-> Critical Methodologies*, 16(2), 141–150.

Thomson, J. and Davies, B. 2019. Becoming with art differently: Entangling matter, thought and love. *Cultural Studies <-> Critical Methodologies*, 19(6), 399–408. DOI: 10.1177/1532708619830123, 1–10.

Wyatt, J. and Davies, B. 2011. Ethics. In J. Wyatt, K. Gale, S. Gannon and B. Davies, (eds.), *Deleuze and Collaborative Writing. An Immanent Plane of Composition*. New York: Peter Lang, 105–129.

3

FINDING AND FOSTERING THE CONDITIONS OF CREATIVE PRODUCTION

In which I introduce Deleuzian transcendental empiricism as a way of thinking/doing new materialist research. I introduce the distinction between Deleuze's and Guattari's interdependent concepts of ambulatory and royal-legal research and link them to Bergson's lines of ascent and descent. To mobilise these ideas/practices, I draw on moments/movements of being/becoming in my own childhood, and in the childhoods of children that I, and others, have encountered in preschools.

In Chapter 2, I explored the possibility of listening to the vital materiality of oneself (never one or self) in intra-action with the vital materiality of the more-than-human world. I drew on the concept of emergent listening to look for ways to interrupt the habituated striations of unquestioned human dominance of the more-than-human world. I was interested in the possibility of generating a sensuous enchantment with that world. In this chapter I explore Deleuzian transcendental empiricism as a way of thinking/doing new materialist research.

Transcendental empiricism

Deleuze makes a radical break with those habituated ways of thinking about human life that depend on "self– consciousness, memory, and personal identity" (Rajchman, 2005: 8). He searches for ways of breaking out into a wilder sort of empiricism, which he calls transcendental empiricism, and which focuses on the movement between beings-becomings that generate increases and decreases in power:

> There is something wild and powerful in this transcendental empiricism that is of course not the element of sensation (simple empiricism), for sensation is only a break within the flow of absolute consciousness. It is, rather, however

> close two sensations may be, the passage from one to the other as becoming, as increase or decrease in power (virtual quantity).
>
> (Deleuze, 2005: 25)

In this break with habituated thought there are two central propositions (Smith and Protevi, forthcoming: np; emphasis added):

> (1) the abstract (e.g. "subject," "object," "State," the "whole," and so on) does not explain, but *must itself be explained*; and (2) the aim of philosophy is not to rediscover the eternal or the universal, but to *find the singular conditions* under which something new is produced.

Deleuze's interest is in "*finding and fostering the conditions of creative production*" (Smith and Protevi, forthcoming: np; emphasis added). He was interested in making, remaking and the unmaking of concepts that go to work "along a moving horizon, from an always decentred centre, from an always displaced periphery which repeats and differenciates them" (Deleuze, 2004: xix).

By de-centring the gaze of the researcher and of individualised subjects, and by keeping hold of the understanding that everything is in motion, Deleuze opens the way to comprehending the apparent paradox that everything repeats itself and at the same time differenciates itself – not differentiating by way of contrast, but in a continuous process of becoming different. The researcher is *of* that world that goes on repeating itself, and yet becoming different. Our own possibilities of knowing in being are opened up through the work we do. We work with our own bodies, our own embeddedness in stratified, codified realities, in order to find and foster the conditions of creative production.

Barad and Bennett also contribute to our capacity to think of our bodies as multiple and intra-active. There were times when I was writing Chapter 2, as I was trying to articulate my embeddedness in the pond assemblage, that I thought readers would think I was mad. And indeed moving out into this unmapped space of transcendental empiricism is not without its dangers. Deleuze both celebrates and cautions against the dangers of what is "wild and powerful in this transcendental empiricism" (Deleuze, 2005: 25).

In everyday life there are hours of the day, and there are days, even weeks and months, where we are carried along by the familiar fabric of life that is un-noteworthy and characterised by routine, by repetitions, and by habituated thoughts and practices. We have all, in 2020, become much more aware of those habituations and our dependence on them as we struggle to adapt to isolating ourselves in response to the coronavirus pandemic. We have lost those thoughtless, comforting days. For some of us, who were miserable in those repetitions, the shutting down can be a welcome relief. For others it is a nightmare.

Transcendental empiricism, too, may confuse and confront as it opens the possibility of leaving the predictable order behind. It awakens and enlivens the senses, opening up a form of reason that is attuned to difference and differenciation. Rather than the bland comfort of the already known, it opens us to intensity, as it engages us in a movement beyond representation and the dualistic pillars of Enlightenment thought:

> This empiricism teaches us a strange "reason", that of the multiple, chaos and difference (nomadic distributions, crowned anarchies) ... The world is neither finite nor infinite as representation would have it: it is completed and unlimited.
> (Deleuze, 2004: 69)

Completed *and* unlimited. Deleuze challenges us, again and again, to hold together what we thought could only be held apart.

I have assembled the following propositions from Deleuze's reflections on a transcendental empiricism, and from Barad's thoughts about diffraction. I draw too from Deleuze and Guattari, and from Bergson to inform the principles of this new materialist methodology:

> The "material and the discursive are mutually implicated" (Barad, 2003: 812);
> The powers of action, intra-action, locution and thought are intimately entangled and emergent;
> Assemblages, in their multiplicity, act on "semiotic, material and social flows simultaneously" (Deleuze and Guattari, 1987: 22–23);
> The duration of the world depends on "invention, the creation of forms, the continual elaboration of the absolutely new" (Bergson, 1998: 11);
> Too wildly de-stratifying may be dangerous (Deleuze and Guattari, 1987: 60);
> Movement is everywhere and nothing stays the same;
> Researchers are *of* the world rather than *in* it, and they are not at all what they thought they were – not beings with identity, or even subjects, but *becomings* that are intricately entangled with others, human and more-than-human;
> Researchers are immanent becomings, whose sense and senses are enlivened in their openness to the other;
> The conceptual possibilities opened up in new materialist thought up-end the habituated, comfortable clichés we've lived with until now;
> Researchers need new strategies for inventing with language and, as I will explore here, with art;
> A new form of response-ability is demanded of us in everything we do.

An answer offered by Deleuze and Guattari to the question of how to proceed with a transcendental empiricism begins with lodging yourself on a 'stratum', where strata are understood in terms of their "giving form to matters, of imprisoning intensities or locking singularities into systems of resonance or redundancy ... organizing them into molar aggregates ... They operate by coding and territorialization upon the earth" (Deleuze and Guattari, 1987: 40). Once lodged on a particular stratum, they suggest, launch yourself into experimenting with the opportunities it offers, and into creating within it a space that is new. Examine the deeper assemblage and the ways you are held by it – and then gently begin to tip it over.

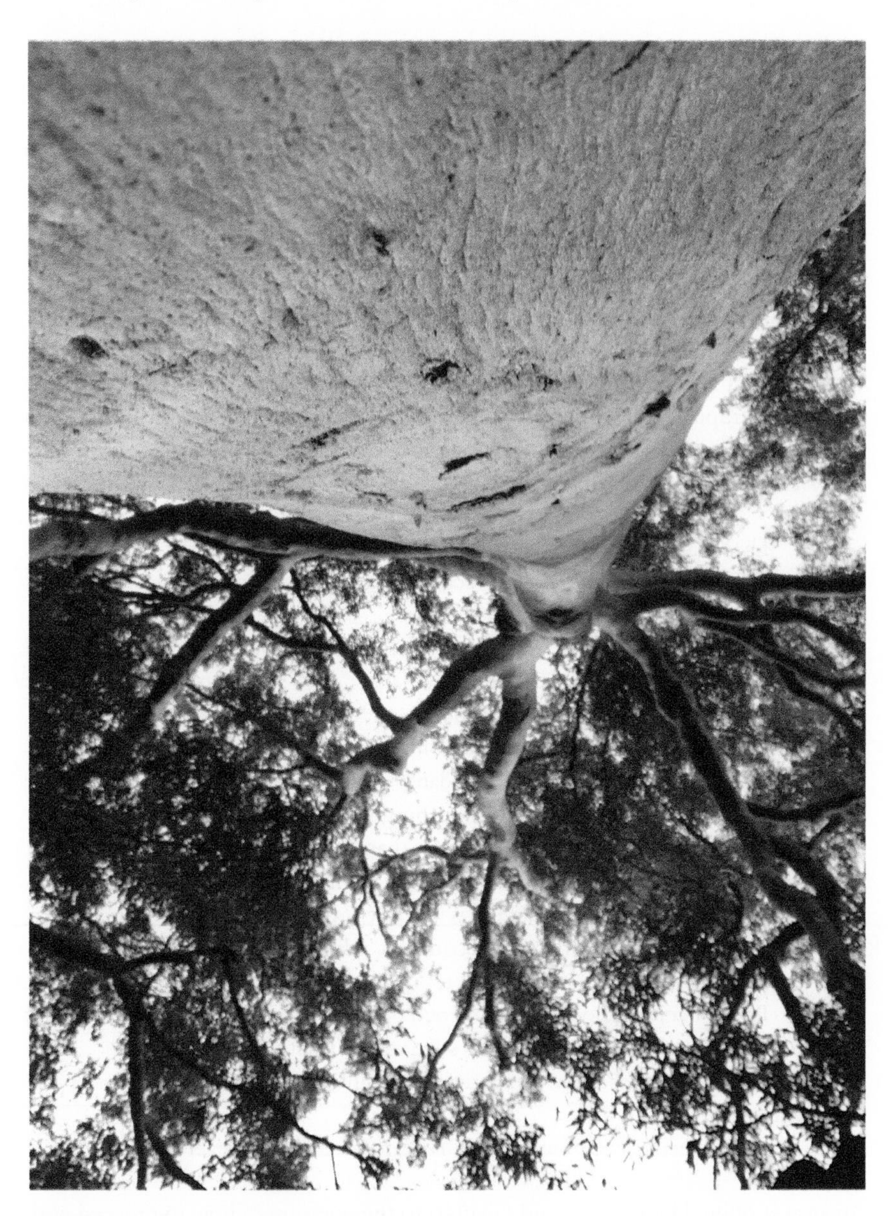

FIGURE 3.1 Gently tip the assemblage.
The Royal Botanic Garden, Sydney. Photograph by Bronwyn Davies, 2020.

> This is how it should be done: Lodge yourself on a stratum, experiment with the opportunities it offers, find an advantageous place on it, find potential movements of deterritorialization, possible lines of flight, experience them, produce flow conjunctions here and there, try out continuums of intensities segment by segment, have a small plot of new land at all times ... We are in a

> social formation; first see how it is stratified for us and in us and at the place where we are; then descend from the strata to the deeper assemblage within which we are held; gently tip the assemblage …
>
> (Deleuze and Guattari, 1987: 161)

In Chapter 1, I lodged myself on the familiar, habituated stratum of grief over a lost friendship, and through an experimental sympoietic form of writing found something new, both conceptually and materially, dislodging the grief and whatever it was that had held me there. This was not simply a matter of generating a singular movement that brought with it an increase in power (it did that), but also a working with that movement to open up new thought. In Chapter 2, I lodged myself in a mother–son stratum and sought to de-territorialise the tedious repetitions in which mother–son were caught up. I de-centred 'myself' in the process, opening myself up to a life much bigger than myself, where I was not simply one and self, as I might have imagined, but conscious of being self-tree-pond-light – our particles interchanged in an immanent singularity.

In such de-territorialising movements, the strata we are held in, that we are implicated in, cannot simply be ignored or overcome. They must be examined closely and carefully, and the work of opening them up to difference (opening ourselves in the process) must proceed carefully as we move toward the plane of consisting; that is, the plane that cuts across all multiplicities, intersecting them "in order to bring into coexistence any number of multiplicities, with any number of dimensions" (Deleuze and Guattari, 1987: 251). (The usual translation for this plane is the plane of consistency, but I think it makes more sense to call it a plane of consisting.)

The multiplicities coexist. It is never a matter of either/or – it is always *and*. Transcendental empiricism does not set out to replace one stratified world with another. *It finds what holds us, in all its variability.* Then, through a close examination of the flows and conjunctions in which we are entangled, we generate new concepts, new ways of knowing in being; we tip things, and ourselves, up, and we open ourselves to the co-existing multiplicities, fostering the conditions of creative production.

What we are used to thinking of as ourselves will be revealed as a "connection of desires, conjunction of flows, continuum of intensities (and as a) … collectivity (assembling elements, things, plants, animals, tools, people, powers, and fragments of all of these … crossing thresholds)" (Deleuze and Guattari, 1987: 161). The sense of oneself as a coherent organism will be (momentarily) abandoned in favour of an openness to those conjunctions and flows, to the collectivities in which we are enfolded and unfolded, mantled and dismantled – and in favour of the materiality of being/becoming human and more-than-human.

> We are made of contracted water, earth, light, air – not merely prior to the recognition or representation of these, but prior to their being sensed. Every organism, in its receptive and perceptual elements, but also in its

> viscera, is a sum of contractions, of retentions and expectations. At the level of this primary vital sensibility, the lived present constitutes a past and a future in time.
>
> (Deleuze, 2004: 93)

This self as multiple and emergent in its responsiveness is not a totalising letting go of ourselves as a coherent organism. That could indeed be the way of madness. We must *also* hold on to a sense of ourselves, since we cannot do otherwise, given our entanglement in dominant realities. Furthermore, Deleuze and Guattari say, we must hold, not totally, but sufficiently, to the *craft,* or skill and dexterity, of researching, which they liken to the craft of surveyors:

> Dismantling the organism has never meant killing yourself, but rather opening the body to connections that presuppose an entire assemblage, circuits, conjunctions, levels and thresholds, passages and distributions of intensity, and territories and deterritorializations *measured with the craft of a surveyor* ... You have to keep enough of the organism for it to reform each dawn; and you have to keep small supplies of signifiance [meaning-making] and subjectification, if only to turn them against their own systems when the circumstances demand it, when things, persons, even situations, force you to; and you have to keep small rations of subjectivity in sufficient quantity to enable you to respond to the dominant reality.
>
> (Deleuze and Guattari, 1987: 160; emphasis added)

Deleuzian transcendental empiricism envisages itself in marked contrast with those familiar empirical methods based on a standard set of assumptions that work with fixed categories and standardised practices. Researchers in that standardised empiricism stand apart from and above the material and semiotic subjects they research; they impose pre-existing meanings on them, all the while claiming that method precludes or obviates any need for theory.

Transcendental empiricism, and new materialist methodology more broadly, open up, in contrast, an exploration of becoming through immanence, where "[i]mmanence refers to the specificity or singularity of a thing; not to what can be made to fit into a pre-existent abstraction" (Coleman and Ringrose, 2013: 10):

> The life of the individual gives way to an impersonal and yet singular life that releases a pure event freed from the accidents of internal and external life, that is, from the subjectivity and objectivity of what happens ... It is a haecceity no longer of individuation but of singularization: a life of pure immanence.
>
> (Deleuze, 2005: 28–29)

This, then, is life's magic: its moments of *haecceity*, its release from the strata, no longer differentiated from the world, but of the world, becoming different from what one was – becoming wave or becoming horizon:

> A haecceity is a moment of pure speed and intensity (an individuation) – like when a swimming body becomes-wave and is momentarily suspended in nothing but an intensity of forces and rhythms. Or like when body becomes-horizon such that it feels only the interplay between curves and surfaces and knows nothing of here and there, observer and observed.
>
> (Halsey, 2007: 146)

Royal-legal and ambulatory research

Returning, then, to the thought that everything is both completed and unlimited, Deleuze and Guattari examine the contrary powers and forces within the research act – those that conserve the way things are done and the way they are spoken about, and those that tap into the emergent possibilities of the not-yet-known. These contrary forces territorialise and re-territorialise, thus holding things the same, and they de-territorialise. These contrary forces Deleuze and Guattari call royal-legal and ambulatory. Royal legal research, like Bergson's line of descent, draws on established concepts and practices – the way things are done, regulated, controlled. Ambulatory thought is emergent and creative. Royal-legal thought territorialises and re-territorialises. Ambulatory thought expands the subject to be researched, develops new concepts, moves outside disciplinary boundaries. It de-territorialises the already known.

Territorialising movements stabilise and normalise; they de-fuse any wayward new thinking, reducing it to fit within already known and established knowledges. Ambulatory research *de*-stabilises; it *follows* the material-semiotic flow of events:

> The ideal of reproduction, deduction, or induction, is part of royal science, at all times and in all places, and treats differences of time and place as so many variables, the constant form of which is extracted precisely by the law ... Reproducing implies the permanence of a fixed point of *view* that is external to what is reproduced ... But following is something different from the ideal of reproduction ... One is obliged to follow when one is in search of the "singularities" of a matter
>
> (Deleuze and Guattari, 1987: 372)

The relationship with the earth changes radically with each of these approaches: "with the legal model one is constantly reterritorializing around a point of view, on a domain, according to a set of constant relations; but with the ambulant model, the process of deterritorialization constitutes and extends the territory itself" (Deleuze and Guattari, 1987: 372).

As with any binary pair, the royal-legal and the ambulatory modes of thought depend on each other. The royal-legal is the dominant one of the pair, but it cannot do without the other – the creative and inventive thinking-in-doing. In a transcendental empiricism or new materialist methodology the ambulatory method becomes dominant, while also depending on the existence of the familiar order (both to draw on, *and* to use in defining what it is not). The inquiries I cite here, with preschool children, mobilise the familiar crafts of observation and interview, which royal-legal administrators and guardians recognise. Yet the lines of flight that open up new ways of thinking are in part already *in* the material, *in* the unstructured interviews, for example, and in the attention to difference; further, the children's thinking and doing is diffracted with new materialist concepts, opening up, in lines of flight, the possibility of seeing the material, and the worlds it opens up, quite differently.

The royal-legal mode has similarities to capitalism and its way of depending on creativity while its administrative/economic arm, neoliberal managerialism, mobilises an obsessive desire to order and control productivity – thus killing off its creativity. In Bergson's terms, the royal-legal mode is a line of *descent*, which holds everything safe and the same. Ethics in the institutionalised line of descent is about legal protection of the institution from those "others" who are being researched, the subtext being that they are inevitably being manipulated and exploited, and thus in a position to sue the institution that supported whatever the research was. Institutional ethics offers, in self-protection, the structuring of research and the formalisation of the ethics approval process. While it is in the ambulatory or lines of *ascent* that the new emerges, institutional ethics is wary of what lies outside the strata from whence its regulation and control take their meaning and power.

The work of ambulatory thought/feeling/actions is to mobilise new concepts, new provocations, new possibilities for expanding thought, feeling, and action. That expansion takes place in "the indefinite time of the event, the floating time that knows only speeds and continually divides that which transpires into an already-there that is at the same time not-yet-here, a simultaneous too-late and too-early, something that is both going to happen and has just happened" (Deleuze and Guattari, 1987: 262). Back and forth. There and not-there. A process that can't be predicted and controlled.

Ambulatory research is kin to Barad's diffractive methodology, which "does not fix what is the object and what is the subject in advance … diffraction involves reading insights through one another in ways that help illuminate differences as they emerge: how different differences get made, what gets excluded, and how these exclusions matter" (Barad, 2007: 30). For Barad, diffractive research involves "being attentive to how differences get made and what the effects of these differences are … [it is] predicated on a relational ontology, an ongoing process in which matter and meaning are co-constituted" (Bozalek and Zembylas, 2017: 112).

Children's lives

In the second half of this chapter, I turn to events involving children that I have written about elsewhere, and open them up again in this space of new materialist, ambulatory methodology. As I have argued elsewhere (Davies, 2016), new materialism does not make a radical break with poststructuralism. My preschool and gender studies have strong continuities with Deleuze's transcendental empiricism.

In the late 1980s and 1990s I hung out in a number of preschools in Australia and Japan. I made notes on encounters I had with the children, I audio-recorded conversations with them about the feminist stories that I (and the Japanese students) read to them, and, when funding permitted, I made video-recordings of the children at play (Davies, 1989; Davies and Kasama, 2004).

Geoffrey was a slight, tow-headed four-year-old in one of the Australian preschools (Davies, 1989). He was not a member of the dominant boys' group, and he could sometimes be seen playing alone. One morning he came into the home corner when no one else was there and made a beeline for the dressing up cupboard. There he selected a black velvet skirt which he pulled on over his trousers. The skirt was gathered at the waist and billowed out around his ankles as he twirled around with obvious pleasure in his immanent liveliness – boy-becoming-skirt and skirt-becoming-boy. A smaller boy came into the home corner and tackled Geoffrey to the ground, pinning him down. Geoffrey fought back but his feet were tangled in the black velvet skirt – that was no longer gorgeous. He yelled at the smaller boy "You're yucky, you made me (—)". He disentangled himself from the arms and legs of the other boy and from the skirt which had become his shackle. He stood up, ripped off the skirt and threw it to the ground, where it lay abject and lifeless. "Now I've got more pants on" he yelled, kicking the smaller boy, who cowered away from the furious legs. Tearful, the smaller boy scrambled up off the floor and ran away.

On another day Geoffrey went into the home corner when Catherine and a small boy, John, were playing with the dolls. John was "ironing" the dolls' clothes. Catherine said to Geoffrey "You be the father", but Geoffrey refused that offer, announcing that he was a fireman.

He put on a fire-fighter's helmet, and another boy joined him, putting on the second helmet. The two boys expanded into their new fire-fighter powers, helmet becoming boy and boy becoming helmet. Then Geoffrey chose a cloth that would stand for the flames he would fight. He flapped the cloth, which in his boy-helmet's hands had taken on new powers. He told the girls he could save them from the fire, and also that his fire could destroy them. It had seemed a small abject piece of cloth, but it held extraordinary power in the firefighter-girl assemblage. The two boys went off to fight the fire. Over the next hour this evolved into the boys threatening the girls with fire, and the girls running into the home corner squealing "Quick, let's hide."

The technician videotaping the home corner was so provoked by this repeated scenario that she asked the girls why they couldn't be firefighters too. The girls pondered this for a while, discussing the fact that the boys were wearing the only helmets. Then they dressed their dollies with hats that might pass for helmets, and, putting them in their prams, went off to fight the fire. Very soon they ran back into the home corner, shocked, and crying "The boys burned our babies!"

Before long the original drama had reinstated itself. Geoffrey and his friend were chasing the girls with fire, and the girls were laughing and squealing "Quick, let's hide." The camera catches a look of complete victory and delight written all over Geoffrey's face as he chases the girls into the home corner, flapping his small piece of cloth.

Deleuze (2005: 30) observes of moments like Geoffrey's in this event: "Small children, through all their sufferings and weaknesses, are infused with an immanent life that is pure power and even bliss." This is not a story about who Geoffrey was or would become. Rather it is an expression of the way a life "is always the index of a multiplicity: an event, a singularity, a life" (Deleuze, 2005: 30). The multiplicity that Geoffrey's life is immanent within, holds both a playful transgendering, and acts of horrific, gendered violence. In 2020, it is particularly chilling revisiting these encounters with Geoffrey. It is three decades since Geoffrey was at preschool. At the time of writing, the news in Australia is full of the story of an estranged husband who set fire to his wife and three small children, killing them all, and then killed himself.

At the time I conducted these studies, the royal-legal doctrine had been being challenged in educational studies for a decade, though not with preschool children. In the early 1980s I had broken with the royal-legal mode in my study of primary school children (Davies, 1982); at the time it was regarded as inconceivable that primary school children would have anything valuable to say about their education. Less than a decade later, when I decided to interview preschool children, I was once again told that they would have nothing of value to say – they must remain objects of our gaze and should not be confused with fully-fledged human beings with agency. Gender was to be explained through sex-role socialisation theory which construed children as passive recipients of the sexist social and linguistic practices of parents, teachers and authors.

Luckily for me, significant papers and books were just beginning to emerge that drew on poststructuralist theory (for example, Weedon, 1987; Henriques et al., 1984), making a radical break with the royal-legal thinking of sex-role socialisation theory. When I first analysed the encounters with Geoffrey, I was intrigued by what I called category-maintenance work. The children's breaks with the gender binary were policed not by adults, but by each other. It was the children who worked on each other to keep the categories of male and female intact, as binaries. My research became an exploration of the gender order inside of which the children lived their bodies.

In the late 1980s, the gender binary was evident everywhere, in the clothes adults and children wore, in the way they spoke, in domestic work, in employment patterns, in the allocation of power. It was, at the same time, being challenged by feminist interventions in those assemblages. My studies had been inspired by the question: *Why does gender matter so much*? It was a question that weighed on me after I had fought my university through the NSW Anti-Discrimination Tribunal, in a fight that lasted for two years, for the right, as a woman, to tenured employment.

Coming to this same material in 2020 with the emergence of new materialism's ambulatory approach to research, I am curious to look again at the ways the children worked and played within the forces and counter-forces of the gender assemblage, in which the binary was dominant and yet also being questioned. What I see is children experimenting with and immanent within lines of ascent – in which Geoffrey could, for example, intra-act with, and become one with a gorgeous black velvet skirt, and the girls could entertain the idea of being heroes *with* the boys, rather than their victims. I am pained now, as I was back then, when I witnessed the ways in which they were forcefully caught back into the lines of descent through which the gendered strata were maintained. In their play they de-territorialised the gender binary and re-territorialised it. It is the play of power in acts of becoming that are mobilised in between one and another that is interesting now; the gender binary was maintained as an apparently totalised state of things even while the children were immanent within and between multiplicities:

> States of things are neither unities nor totalities, but *multiplicities* ... The essential thing, from the point of view of empiricism, is the noun multiplicity, which designates a set of lines or dimensions which are irreducible to one another. Every "thing" is made up in this way. Of course a multiplicity includes focuses of unification, centres of totalization, points of subjectivation, but as factors which can prevent its growth and stop its lines ... In a multiplicity what counts are not the terms or the elements, but what there is 'between', the between, a set of relations which are not separable from each other.
>
> (Deleuze and Parnet, 1987: vii–viii)

The fluidity of the children's engagement in the gender assemblage did not always coincide with the views of the adults in their lives, or the media, or the books they read. The children talked about the importance of obeying their parents, for example, when they told you how to get your gender right. They also talked about teasing others who did not do their gender right according to the binary order. George was a boy who sometimes played in the home corner and sometimes wore capes and skirts. In our discussion about the character Oliver, in *Oliver Button Is a Sissy* (de Paola, 1981), George said it was OK for Oliver to do all the things he did, such as picking flowers and dressing up. But he must not play with paper dolls, since only girls can do that. Although George expressed a more open attitude to gender than Oliver Button's father or the children in the story, who teased Oliver, at the end of our conversation he claimed that no matter what, fathers are the ones who are always right:

> (OK. What about dressing up? Is that a girl thing or a boy thing or both?) Both. (Uh huh. Right. But his dad doesn't think that does he? His dad thinks they're all girl things?) Yes. (Is his dad right or wrong?) Right. (His dad's right?) Yep. (Why is his dad right? 'cause we think they're girl things *and* boy things but his dad thinks they're just girl things. And do you think that his dad's right?) Yes. (So he disagrees with us and he's right?) Yeah. (Well I think we're right. I think that boys can do those things … So are daddies right all the time?) Yeah … (So can mummies be wrong?) Yep. (Can daddies be wrong?) No. They can be right. (They can be right? And they can't be wrong?) Uh uh. George shakes his head.
>
> (Davies, 1989: 131–132)

So, what is added to, or changed from, my earlier poststructuralist analysis with the benefit of this transcendental empiricist, and new materialist lens?

Instead of thinking in terms of a dominant discourse being reasserted and overwhelming the subordinate feminist discourse, the movements in between and among discourses can be seen as more fluid and multiple – more dynamic, and they can be seen as creative lines of ascent that de-territorialise the gender order and that will in turn be re-territorialised. Lives and genders are territorialised and de-territorialised, sometimes within the same event; the apparently intractable strata are in fact constantly changing. As Feely (2019: 6) observes:

> we can identify and arrange an assemblage's components along a *material/semiotic continuum;* map *flows* of heterogeneous substances within the assemblage; and consider forces of continuity and change within the assemblage along a deterritorialization/reterritorialization continuum.

In his entanglement with the smaller boy Geoffrey discovered the risk of a loss of power that his experimentation involved. His line of flight had established a pleasurable relation between his moving body and the texture and movement of the skirt. But this experiment opened him up to an attack from a boy who would not usually have dared to fight him. That attack made Geoffrey's body weak and tearful. In re-establishing the masculine power that he had lost, Geoffrey re-territorialised his body as dominant by casting the black velvet skirt on to the floor, reclaiming his masculinity in intra-action with his pants, turning his tears into affective rage. Kicking his foe again and again, he turned the smaller boy into a cowering and fearful other who could be subdued.

Since there were only two fire-fighter helmets in the home corner, the girls generated their line of flight as firefighters by dressing their dolls with hats. This time Geoffrey was the one to violently reject the girls' experiment in sharing power. In both cases, the line of ascent shifted rapidly back into a line of descent – and into the repetition of familiar gendered lines – lines that took no thought and needed no practice, were re-established.

In the decades since my preschool children and gender studies, there have been multiple feminist interventions in the state of things. Gender can be both totalised through particular strata *and* be open to movement, then, now and in the future.

Renold and Mellor (2013: 34–35) videotaped two preschool children playing together, territorialising the space between them in gendered terms, and deterritorialising it at the same time. I explore this intra-action at length in part because it suggests a significant loosening of the gender order I had observed in the earlier work.

Sophie and Tyler were boyfriend and girlfriend, and in their play together Action Man and Barbie have evident thing-power:

> Sophie and Tyler are sat opposite each other on a soft mat, in the outside play area … Sophie is sat with legs tucked under her. Tyler is squatting. The camera enters the scene as Tyler is turning an Action Man doll over and over. Sophie clutches her Action Man under the arms so that he is standing upright. The Action Man dolls face each other. "Fight again yeah", says Tyler to Sophie. "Yeah", says Sophie. She pushes her Action Man into Tyler's Action Man and he spins the Action Man again. "Fight again, fight again, yeah … fight again". Sophie looks over at Becky who is holding Princess Barbie, and pulls her Action Man away. "What you doin?" says Tyler, "it's better have a fighting man, eh?" Sophie puts her Action Man down by her side. Tyler picks up another Barbie. He pushes the two dolls together, their faces touching, and then throws the Barbie into the doll box. Gesturing with the Action Man he says again, "Get the man … get the man". Sophie shakes her head. "You have to … you have to". She shakes her head again. Tyler picks up her Action Man and thrusts it into her hands, saying "get it, get … it". She doesn't move. "You have to … you have to". He is now holding the two Action men and shouts, "YOU HAVE TO, YOU HAVE TO". Sophie shakes her head, and raises her shoulders up and down. He reaches into the doll box, "you want this? You want a girl?" "Yeah", says Sophie, smiling. She takes the Princess Barbie. She looks at the doll, they face each other, and she turns the doll around to face Tyler's Action Man. "Let's have a fight", Tyler says, as Action Man does a somersault. "Yes", says Sophie. She holds Princess Barbie's legs with two hands and Barbie head-butts Action Man, sending him spinning to the ground. She hits him again, and again and again.
>
> (Renold and Mellor, 2013: 34–35)

Sophie and Tyler begin their play, each with an Action Man, each engaging in what Action Men do – taking the lead in their play from the Action Men. Then Sophie notices Becky, who is holding Princess Barbie, and the event changes. Princess Barbie has interrupted – interfered with – the Action Men's power. There is now a line of force in between the two girls and Princess Barbie. The desirability of this particular Barbie doll is palpable. It takes Tyler a while to tune into this new dynamic; he gives way to it. The thing-power of Princess Barbie then becomes greater than the thing-power of Action Man. The gender dynamic that Tyler mobilised in ordering Sophie to fight, even shouting at her, gave way to a Sophie-Princess Barbie thing-power, which included her power to demolish Tyler-Action Man again and again.

Curiously Tyler-Action Man does not object. The important thing is the event of the staged fight. The fight is the thing – win or lose. And Sophie-Barbie both enters into Tyler-Action Man's idea of what matters while simultaneously establishing the superior power of Sophie-Barbie.

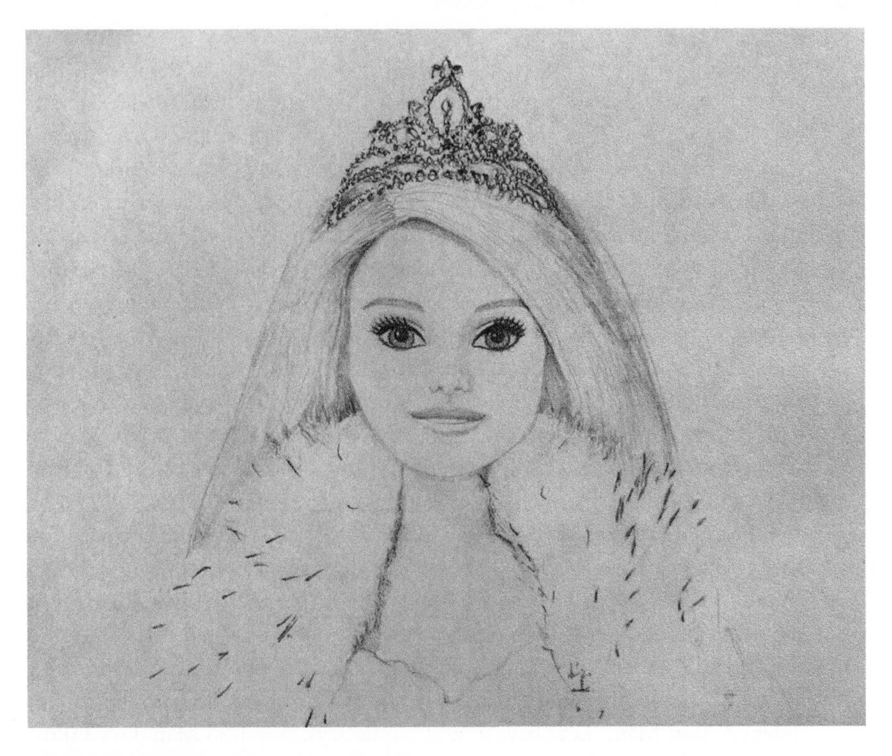

FIGURE 3.2 Jody Thomson, *Princess Barbie*. Pencil on paper (2020).

Language, and in particular conventional language forms, in which royal-legal research has traditionally been reported, is insufficient for new materialist work. The crafts of interview and observation, of transcription, can be mobilised as recognisable forms for doing inquiry, though the royal-legal apparatus would have great difficulty with open-ended interviews and observations in which the observers are present and involved. The old crafts need major modifications, and new crafts need to be invented. We must draw also on poetry, art and literature to open up our capacities to know and to be differently – to open up our capacity for sympathy and response-ability. Art "produces sensations, affects, intensities as its mode of addressing problems" (Grosz, 2008: 1–2). The nonhuman world has different modes of communication: the black velvet skirt, Action Man, Barbie, firefighter helmets, a piece of cloth; each communicates, each is, in a sense an affective work of art, communicating lines of flight, connecting with bodies, generating new assemblages: Geoffrey becomes the gorgeous black velvet skirt, the piece of cloth becomes fire, the boys become helmets become fire-fighters, the dolls and their hats become fire-fighters. Sophie-Barbie takes on sufficient power to defeat an ascendant and annoyingly persistent Action Man. What becomes evident in this new materialist analysis is the way "the entire world tries to speak itself out ... to show itself, to open itself, that is, to declare itself for what it is ... In fact, the entire world has never stopped looking for an expression" (Nancy, 2017: 115). In taking up an ambulatory approach we must learn to listen with all our senses to that which we do not yet know how to hear:

> To be listening is thus to enter into tension and to be on the lookout for a relation to self: not, it should be emphasized, a relationship to "me" (the supposedly given subject), or the "self" of the other (the speaker, the musician, also supposedly given, with his subjectivity), but to the relationship in self, so to speak, as it forms a "self" or a "to itself" in general ... [where] "self" is precisely nothing available (substantial or subsistent) to which one can be "present," but precisely the resonance of a return [renvoi] ... a reality consequently indissociably "mine" and "other,"singular" and "plural," as much as it is "material" and spiritual and "signifying" and "a-signifying."
>
> (Nancy, 2007: 12)

To listen in this way, to be open to the chaos of events, is a painful and sometimes rapturous necessity of coming to compose something new. We must place ourselves on the plane of composition, which:

> cuts across and thus plunges into, filters and coheres chaos through the coming into being of sensation [and] is thus both an immersion in chaos but also a mode of disruption and ordering of chaos through the extraction of that which life can glean for itself and its own intensification from this whirling complexity – sensations, affects, percepts, intensities – blocs of bodily becoming that always co-evolve with blocs of becoming of matter or events.
>
> (Grosz, 2008: 9)

Lines of descent in preschools are not unlike thinking/feeling/doing in the royal-legal mode of research. They draw on already known concepts and possibilities, reiterating and affirming aspects of the territory that has been laid down again and again. The royal-legal mode of research appeals to "the striated space of the cogito universalis and draws a path that must be followed from one point to another" (Deleuze and Guattari, 1987: 377). "YOU HAVE TO, YOU HAVE TO," shouts Tyler. Only daddies can be right, asserts George. And from Geoffrey: I will burn your babies if you disrupt the gender binary in which I am dominant.

The movement of new thought-feeling-action requires a space–time in which the form or structure has in it room for movement. Such space, Deleuze and Guattari call smooth space. It is not structured by the cogito universalis: "there is no possible method, no conceivable reproduction, but only relays, intermezzos, resurgences" (Deleuze and Guattari, 1987: 377). In contemplating the children at play, I have made observable some of those relays, intermezzos and resurgences.

As new materialist researchers we depend on de-territorialising movements that disrupt the conceptual, material and practical striations of familiar territory. Those movements are neither unitary or linear; they form an assemblage, which "in its multiplicity, necessarily acts on semiotic flows, material flows, and social flows simultaneously (independently of any recapitulation that may be made of it in a scientific or theoretical corpus)" (Deleuze and Guattari, 1987: 22–23). The vitality of the research, and of life, depends on being open to those multiple unpredictable flows – to the possibility of wandering off known paths, though the paths are still there; and the fear of going off them may be palpable – the punishment may be brutal.

While there can be said to be no method for working in smooth space other than getting lost in "relays, intermezzos, and resurgences", the already known territory, and the de-territorialising not-yet-known, depend on each other. The lines of ascent with their poetic play among the "relays, intermezzos and resurgences" are life-giving, generating new ways of "knowing in being" (Barad, 2007: 185). The rhythms of the poetic play, following the "semiotic flows, material flows, and social flows" (Deleuze and Guattari, 1987: 22–23) must find their way to "impose" themselves on the lines of descent, where in turn they risk being re-territorialised, though they can never become exactly what they were before.

New materialist research explores the ways human subjects are entangled in others' lines of force, enveloped in multiple, co-existing, co-implicated strata, and constantly in motion, not on a linear trajectory from past to future, nor on a single trajectory from bad to good, and not in search of identities. It is open to the singularities of being and becoming and of the in-between. It dismantles the *cogito universalis,* and it opens up the not-yet-known. It works its way into the space of imagination, inviting us not to fail at the threshold of such binaries such as animate/inanimate and epistemology/ontology. It pulls up the anchors that bind the human imagination to the small ship of individual identity. It opens up the creative impulse and power of ambulatory research, and shifts the ground of royal-legal thinking, however minutely, in each successive mo(ve)ment.

References

Barad, K. 2003. Posthumanist performativity: How matter comes to matter. *Signs: Journal of Women in Culture and Society*, 28(3), 801–831.

Barad, K. 2007. *Meeting the Universe Halfway: Quantum Physics and the Entanglement of Matter and Meaning*. Durham, NC: Duke University Press.

Bergson, H. 1998. *Creative Evolution* (trans. A. Mitchell). Mineola, NY: Dover Publications Inc.

Bozalek, V. and Zembylas, M. 2017. Diffraction or reflection? Sketching the contours of two methodologies in educational research. *International Journal of Qualitative Studies in Education*, 30(2), 111–117. DOI: 10.1080/09518398.2016.1201166.

Coleman, R. and Ringrose, J. 2013. *Introduction*. In R. Coleman and J. Ringrose (eds), *Deleuze and Research Methodologies*. Edinburgh: Edinburgh University Press, 1–22.

Davies, B. 1989. *Frogs and Snails and Feminist Tales. Preschool Children and Gender*. Sydney, NSW: Allen & Unwin.

Davies, B. 2016. Ethics and the new materialism. A brief genealogy of the "post" philosophies in the social sciences. *Discourse Studies in the Cultural Politics of Education*, 39(1), 113–127. http://www.tandfonline.com/doi/full/10.1080/01596306.2016.1234682.

Davies, B. (2017 [1982]) *Life in the Classroom and Playground. The Accounts of Primary School Children*. London: Routledge and Kegan Paul.

Davies, B. 2019. *New Lives in an Old Land. Re-turning to the Colonization of New South Wales through Stories of my Parents and their Ancestors*. Sydney, NSW: Ornythorhynchus Paradoxus Books.

Davies, B. and Kasama, H. 2004. *Gender in Japanese Preschools. Frogs and Snails and Feminist Tales in Japan*. Cresskill, NJ: Hampton Press.

Deleuze, G. 2004. *Difference and Repetition* (trans. P. Patton). London: Continuum.

Deleuze, G. 2005. *Pure Immanence: Essays on a Life* (trans. A. Boyman). New York: Zone.

Deleuze, G. and Guattari, F. 1987. *A Thousand Plateaus: Capitalism and Schizophrenia* (trans. B. Massumi). Minneapolis, MN: University of Minnesota Press.

Deleuze, G. and Parnet, C. 1987. *Dialogues 11 Revised Edition* (trans. H. Tomlinson and B. Habberjam). New York: Columbia University Press.

de Paola, T. 1981. *Oliver Button Is a Sissy*. London: Methuen.

Feely, M. 2019. Assemblage analysis: An experimental new-materialist method for analyzing narrative data. *Qualitative Research*. DOI: 10.1177/1468794119830641, 1–20.

Grosz, E. 2008. *Chaos, Territory, Art: Deleuze and the Framing of the Earth*. New York: Columbia University Press.

Halsey, M. 2007. Molar ecology: What can the (full) body of an eco-tourist do? In A. Hickey-Moody and P. Malins (eds), *Deleuzian Encounters: Studies in Contemporary Social Issues*. Basingstoke: Palgrave Macmillan, 135–150.

Henriques, J., Hollway, W., Urwin, C. and Walkerdine, V. 1984. *Changing the Subject: Psychology, Social Regulation and Subjectivity*. London: Methuen.

Nancy, J.-L. 2007. *Listening* (trans. C. Mandell). New York: Fordham University Press.

Nancy, J.-L. 2017. *The Possibility of a World: Conversations with Pierre-Philippe Jandin* (trans. T. Hollway and F. Mechain). New York: Fordham University Press.

Rajchman, J. 2005. Introduction. In G. Deleuze, *Pure Immanence: Essays on A Life* (trans. A. Boyman). New York: Zone Books, 7–23.

Renold, E. and Mellor, D. 2013. Deleuze and Guattari in the nursery: Towards an ethnographic multi-sensory mapping of gendered bodies and becomings. In R. Coleman and J. Ringrose (eds), *Deleuze and Research Methodologies*. Edinburgh: Edinburgh University Press, 23–41.
Smith, D. and Protevi, J. forthcoming. "Gilles Deleuze". In E. N. Zalta (ed.), *The Stanford Encyclopedia of Philosophy* (Spring 2020 edition), forthcoming URL = https://plato.stanford.edu/archives/spr2020/entries/deleuze/.
Weedon, C. 1987. *Feminist Practice and Poststructuralist Theory*. Oxford: Blackwell.

4

THING-POWER

> In which I focus on the power of things as active agents in the world. I tell a story of a workshop where the participants learned to read others from the space around them and from things they had in their possession. I turn then to an event in my own life which I have written about many times, and created works of art in relation to, and tell it differently through focusing on the power of things.

So far, I have visited, from a number of angles, the conceptual and practical means of freeing ourselves from the isolating Cartesian-Enlightenment version of ourselves as bounded, and ultimately unknowable in our separation from the world. That freeing dissolves identity and opens up the extraordinary singularity of knowing-in-being, or being-in-knowing, of intra-active, multiplicative, emergent subjects. At the same time, I have explored the strata that hold things the same, and the interdependence of those strata with creative lines of flight through which the new emerges. In Chapter 3, I explored Deleuzian conceptual strategies for finding and fostering the conditions of creative production. I drew on childhood events to look at the *movement in between* moments of creativity or opening up of the new, and the strata on which they are lodged, strata that give form to matters "locking singularities into systems of resonance or redundancy … organizing them into molar aggregates … coding and territorialization upon the earth" (Deleuze and Guattari, 1987: 40).

In this chapter I turn again to thing-power: "the curious ability of [apparently] inanimate things to animate, to act, to produce effects dramatic and subtle" (Bennett, 2010: 6). I ponder on where our bodies begin and end. We tend to think of skin as the surface or container of the person within. But life is not lived in that 'container'; lives are intra-active, and there are flows in between humans, and in-between humans and the more-than-human. We are *of* the world, not *in* it. I begin this chapter with the space immediately outside the skin, a space that is not usually visible, though it is tangible.

The workshop

I became fascinated by this space around the body, invisible to my eyes, when I met a masseur whose massages took place in that energy field around my body. The massages were surprisingly calming and soothing in spite of his making no skin contact. And nor did he bother with sound – of music or words to facilitate relaxation.

I enrolled in a weekend workshop he organised, where participants could learn some of the skills he brought to his massage practice. He co-ran the workshop with an older, reclusive friend/colleague, who was presented to the participants as having particular psychic powers, some of which we could learn.

It was the 1980s, a time of great openness to the unknown, before the closing down engineered through the introduction of neoliberal discourses and practices, whose purpose was to create assemblages that brought us all back under control, converting us into separate, vulnerable homo economicus, competing with each other for survival. The psychology degree I had completed back in the 1960s had included psychic powers as part of its investigations. In the 1980s that was an aspect of the discipline that was in process of being closed down to become "part of a lost psychology or a future psychology-yet-to-come, which worked with more relational, distributed, and transsubjective ontologies of personhood" (Blackman, 2015: 32).

In one of the sessions in the workshop we were instructed to choose a partner to work with. The exercise was simple. We would take it in turns to place our hands inside the space behind our partner's back without touching and without words. We would then report what we could feel there. I anticipated that this space would be no more than two centimetres deep, but I could get my hands to move no closer than twenty centimetres from my partner's back. It felt as if there were triangular spikes coming out of his back that were capable of pushing my hands back. When I reported what I had sensed, my partner confessed that he had felt threatened by my coming up behind him – and that he had not wanted me to come any closer. His body's capacity to ward me off was contained in the virtual particles that formed those spikes outside what we normally think of as 'the body'.

Barad observes that "particles no longer take their place in the void; rather they are constitutively entangled with it. As for the void, it is no longer vacuous. It is a loving, breathing indeterminacy of non/being" (Barad, 2015: 156). Perhaps unsurprisingly, my partner's hands did not sense anything in the space behind my back. He could not tune into that space in between; his energy was all directed to holding me apart. Touching is no simple encounter between one set of actual particles and another:

> In an important sense, touch is the primary concern of physics. Its entire history can be understood as a struggle to articulate what touch entails.

> How do particles sense one another? Through direct contact, an ether, action-at-a-distance forces, fields, the exchange of virtual particles? What does the exchange of energy entail? How is a change in motion effected? What is pressure? What is temperature? How does the eye see? How do lenses work? What are the different kinds of forces that particles experience?
>
> (Barad, 2015: 155)

On the second day of the workshop we were asked to bring something with us that we had had close to us. We sat in a circle and each put the thing we had brought into a box that was passed around. We took care not to look at who was putting what into the box. The box was then passed around again and we each drew out an item. I drew out a man's watch. I hadn't met any of the men sitting in the circle prior to the workshop.

We were instructed as follows: Hold the item in both hands, cupped together at the level of your navel. Focus on the item. Close your eyes. Imagine that your brain is like an amoeba, and that it can put out a pseudopod or feeler that reaches down to the object and gently wraps itself around it, encircling it, taking it inside yourself. While your brain thus contains it, use all of your senses to discover what it tells you.

At first, I was sceptical and a little impatient with this exercise, thinking it was rather silly. I was sure nothing was going to happen in-between me and the watch. But I had studied biology and understood the amoeba-like action I was being asked to imagine.

Quite soon a vivid series of images began to unfold.

The setting of those images was the interior of an A frame beach house I had once stayed in with a friend; that friend was at the workshop.

On a small wooden table in the A frame was a jigsaw puzzle. The picture in the puzzle was of two identical snow-covered mountains. At the base of one of the jigsaw mountains was a man with three dogs.

The man was furious because he couldn't choose which mountain to climb.

Astonishingly, he climbed out of the jigsaw and down off the table. He ran out of the A frame on to a path that led down to the beach.

As he ran, his heart was pounding.

As soon as his heart started pounding, I knew whose watch it was – whose heart it was that was pounding. I looked up at him. The pounding of the jigsaw man's heart was the same pounding as that of the heart of the man sitting across from me.

It *was* his watch, he admitted, in the discussion that followed this exercise. But what I had seen, he said, made no sense to him.

The owner of the watch, and the friend with whom I had shared a holiday in the A-frame in which the jigsaw had appeared, unbeknown to me at the time, had just become lovers. She was at the workshop and she had, in a separate exercise, described herself as a mountain.

A year after the workshop she discovered that he had another lover. Until the two women met, they both thought they were in a full-time relationship with the owner of the watch.

He was often absent, but there were reasons for that. He had regularly to go to his farm in the mountains to tend to his three dogs. He was a member of a running club, which often went on weekend-long running excursions, including excursions to the seaside. He created the fiction that he had rented a room in the house of my friend, telling the 'other woman' that he had done so because he sometimes needed to be alone. If he slipped up, forgetting which woman was which, and saying something that didn't make sense, he explained that due to a blow to his head as a child he sometimes became confused. It thus 'made sense' to each woman that he was at home only half of each week. When the two women confronted him, having discovered each other, and pieced together all the bits of the jigsaw of their double lives, he left the scene altogether, running off with another woman, who was a member of his running club.

What is perhaps most interesting in that flow in between me, my friend, the watch and its owner, was that when I held the watch cupped in my hands, much of what I sensed hadn't happened yet. He had only just begun his relationship with my friend, and the women had not yet discovered each other.

Any beginning, Barad says, "is always already threaded through with anticipation of where it is going" (Barad, 2010: 244):

> the past is never left behind, never finished once and for all, and the future is not what will come to be in an unfolding of the present moment; rather the past and the future are enfolded participants in matter's iterative becoming. Becoming is not an unfolding in time, but the inexhaustible dynamism of the enfolding of mattering.
>
> (Barad, 2007: 234)

Deleuze writes about "a life" of a given living subject being everywhere, in particular in the between-times and between-moments, and between a subject and "lived objects":

> A life is everywhere, in all the moments that a given living subject goes through and are measured by given lived objects: an immanent life carrying with it the events or singularities that are merely actualized in subjects and objects. This indefinite life does not itself have moments, close as they may be one to another, but only between-times, between moments; it doesn't come about or come after but offers the immensity of an empty time where one sees the event yet to come and already happened, in the absolute of an immediate consciousness.
>
> (Deleuze, 2005: 29)

It's possible the moment in between me and the watch-owner was one in which he saw only the immensity of an empty time, when all things were yet still possible. Or, perhaps, because his watch told its story in images rather than words, he didn't know how to hear them.

For some readers, this story of thing-power will have been a step too far. Can things really hold so much of us – or work to open up access to each other's lives, past, present and future? Can watches, ponds, black velvet skirts, fire-fighters' helmets, Barbie dolls, Action Men have more relational agency even than that they've been granted in the explorations I've undertaken so far? To open this question out further, it's helpful to mobilise the concept of assemblages.

A note on assemblages

In thinking about thing-power and puzzling over how some thing, that is usually thought of as inanimate, might have agency, it would be easy to slip into thinking about agency in liberal humanist terms. In those terms, agency is an individual's (usually a human individual's) capacity to act on the world and change it, or to hold it the same. And in those terms, things that we think of as inanimate don't and can't have agency. In new materialist terms, in marked contrast, agency is not only to do with an individual's power to affect others, but a matter of matter's response-ability; animate and inanimate beings, human, animal and earth beings, are not alone; rather they are constantly, collectively, affecting and being affected by others within multiple onto-epistemological assemblages: "In an important sense, in a breathtakingly intimate sense, touching, sensing, is what matter does, or rather, what matter is: matter is condensations of response-ability" (Barad, 2015: 161). Matter, including the matter of us, responds, it intra-acts; "the 'I' as a compound of human and nonhuman parts, is continually entering and leaving larger assemblages (ideologies, diets, cultures, technological regimes) made up of other sets of composite or compound bodies" (Bennett, 2012: 256).

Human agency, then, is effected within assemblages that are made up of other humans and other beings, animate, *and* what we usually think of as inanimate: "While the smallest or simplest body or bit may indeed express a vital impetus … an actant never really acts alone. Its efficacy or agency always depends on the collaboration, or interactive interference of many bodies and forces" (Bennett, 2010: 21). Bennett calls this distributive agency.

Thinking diffractively, in this way, material beings can be said to have a vital impetus, and at the same time each body, each thing, is associative, "continuously affecting and being affected by other bodies" (Bennett, 2010: 21). Each of us is thus, necessarily, indeterminate and emergent: "in an important sense, the self is dispersed/diffracted through time and being" (Barad, 2015: 159). We are each, then, not so much subjects or objects but what Spinoza calls a "mode"; that is, we are emergent within shifting relations and assemblages:

> What it means to be a "mode," then, is to form alliances and enter assemblages: it is to mod(e)ify and be modified by others. The process of modification is

> not under the control of any one mode – no mode is an agent in the hierarchical sense. Neither is the process without tension, for each mode vies with and against the (changing) affections of (a changing set of) other modes, all the while being subject to the elements of chance or contingency intrinsic to any encounter.
>
> (Bennett, 2010: 22)

In the following section, I make a new interpretation of an old story, by thinking in terms of the diffractive assemblage of my marriage and its ending.

The end of my marriage

I have written, more than once, the story of my marriage, and, in particular, its violent ending that took place fifty years ago, my writing "spilling blood and life across a dusty page. That's what writing will do" (Bright, 2018: 104). More recently I have explored art-making as a different way into and potentially out of the remembered pain of it (Davies, 2018; Thomson et al., 2018), though I suspect this is an event that can never be ended – lodged as it is in my past which is also my present and future. It is intensely personal and specific, yet it taps into the gender patterns of our social strata in which violence is "accomplished almost instantaneously, like releasing a spring" (Bergson, 1998: 11). One woman a week is murdered by her male partner in Australia. Police are called out to deal with domestic violence more than to any other kind of event (Hill, 2019). And during the coronavirus pandemic, in 2020, the women's shelters have been unable to meet the demand of fleeing women and children.

In one of my ventures into art-making, an image of two birds in a fight to the death took me by surprise. I had not thought of my struggle to protect my life and the lives of my children as a fight to the death, until that image found its way into my creation (Davies, 2018). That strong young woman, just 25 years old at the time of her husband's death, took me by surprise. A number of people, who knew nothing of my marriage, had asked me at the time if I felt guilty after Larry's death. In that line of descent on guilt, one or other is the victim, which means the other is the dominant aggressor. I would have had to position myself as fragile and helpless if I were to avoid that storyline. Instead I launched myself with joy into life, wary even now, though, about the presumption of guilt, which being joyful or strong might plunge me into.

That particular work of art, with its image of two birds fighting, I keep on the table inside my front door. It is made from a shoe box with a hinged lid. The box is painted black and the inside is red. There are images on almost all the surfaces that tell both of entrapment and release. Inside the black box is another smaller gold box that holds inside it a small faded photo of Larry with me and the three children.

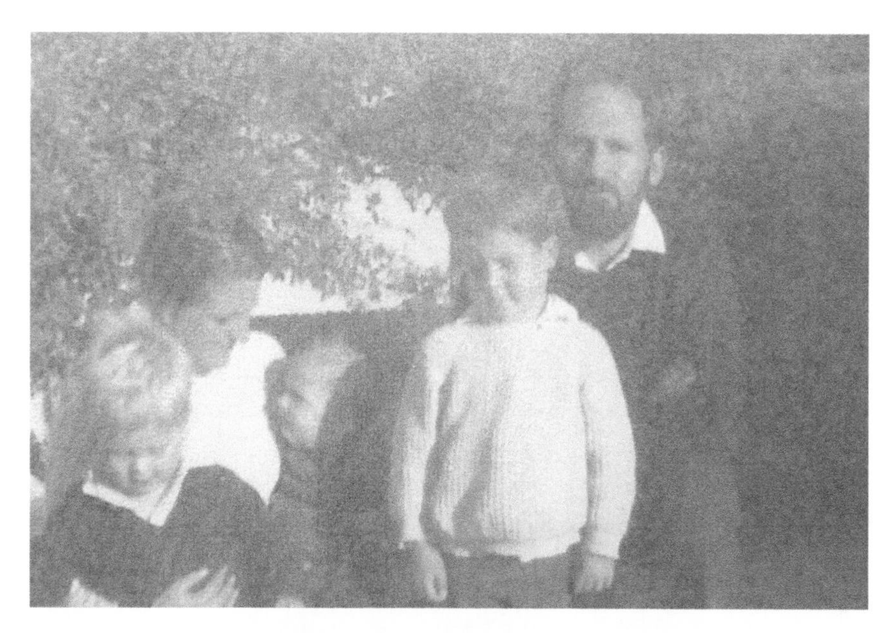

FIGURE 4.1 A year before Larry's death. Bronwyn, Larry and their three children. Tamworth, NSW. Photograph by Norma Davies, 1970.

It was taken by my mother the year before Larry died. The gold box holds him safe, almost tenderly, but it also holds me safe from his violent eruption back into the world, as can happen in my nightmares (Wyatt et al., 2011). The box is not an attempt to represent what was, but a material becoming:

> Art engenders becomings, not imaginative becomings – the elaboration of images and narratives in which a subject might recognize itself, not self-representations, narratives, confessions, testimonies of what is and has been – but material becomings, in which these imponderable universal forces touch and become enveloped in life … in which each exchanges some elements or particles with the other to become more and other.
>
> (Grosz, 2008: 23)

I have been asked why the box sits just there, on the marble table in the foyer of my flat. It has, after all, no particular artistic merit. The thing is, I didn't have a "reason" to put it there. Rather, it settled itself down there. Its imponderable, conflicting forces are contained. Sitting there, in that place, the box emanates a quiet calm. If I open it, however, the violence and the pain can begin to spill out – like Pandora's box.

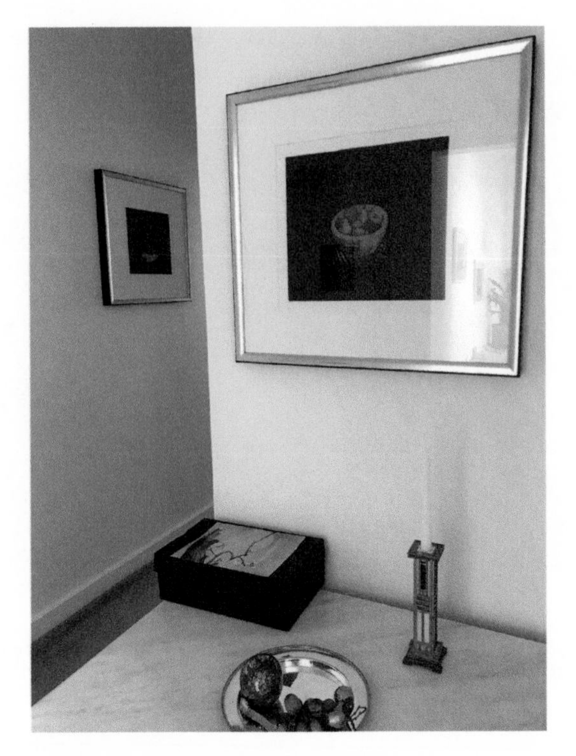

FIGURE 4.2 Bronwyn Davies, Pandora's box.
Photo by Bronwyn Davies, 2020.

What I want to do now, here, is something quite different from the making and keeping of my box. I return to words instead of images, but this time with a new-found focus on the diffractive assemblage of *things* that were at play at the end of my marriage.

Two days before my husband killed himself, I was in the kitchen by the fuel stove, which I was struggling to light. The flue was blocked. As it later turned out, a possum had made his home inside the flue. Larry continually refused to get in a chimney sweep. He couldn't bear the thought of other men in the house.

I needed to empty the ash to help open up whatever draught was possible through the flue. The lock in the back door was stuck. I headed for the front door with the ash, disobeying Larry, who said it must be emptied out the back. He grabbed my arm and tried to force me to go out the back door, saying he would show me how to unlock it. I refused, infuriated by the situation I was caught in. If I did not get his breakfast cooked on time, there would be a disastrous and probably violent scene. The three small children were waiting quietly in the bedroom until he left for work. My brother who had come to stay, against Larry's wishes, was still asleep.

When I came back inside to struggle again with the stove, Larry began to strangle me. Then he stopped. He stopped for no reason that I was aware of. He glanced over his shoulder. He let me go.

My memory of that day contains this unexplained pause. This break. What (in)animate forces were at play? What "individual particles which are seemingly autonomous or independent and yet entangled with each other" (de Freitas, 2017: 747) might have generated such a break?

Some of the other things with power or agency involved in that event were the prisons, where Larry had spent his teenage years and early adulthood, the hidden key to the trunk with the butchering implements inside it, his teeth, and the markings on his body, inflecting him with his own ex-prisoner particularity. Larry and I were singular beings, but we were also emergent in the diffractive/diffracting assemblage of our marriage. Immediately after the break, the pause, neither of us spoke, and the hidden key to the trunk that contained the butchering implements, became a wildly vibrating thing which I was aware could turn this event into a different and bloody event – different from the one it turned out to be.

I was slumped on the bench by the stove where Larry had dropped me. As he paced through the house, I knew without words being spoken, that he was looking for the key. I concentrated on not visualising where it was, on not setting up a flow between myself and the key; I was afraid that if I thought of it in its hiding place, that place would leap from my mind's eye to his. I concentrated on thinking of other places in the house – anywhere except where the key was. Larry had asked me months before to hide the key to the trunk, because he could not, in his view, be trusted with access to the butchering knives and cleaver. He had bought those implements so we could butcher our own meat. When we bought a half-beast, he would go outside while I retrieved the key from its hiding place. When the meat was cut and wrapped and placed in the freezer, and the implements were cleaned and locked in the trunk, Larry would go outside again and water his vegetable garden while I re-hid the key.

The narrative of a violent man who inexplicably stopped strangling his wife is interrupted with this detail. This is a man afraid of his own violence, who had sought to protect himself and others from it. On that morning, I realise now, he did not ask me where the key was. He did, and did not, want that key and the mayhem it could unleash. While I sat there on the bench by the unlit stove and Larry searched for the key, there was a tangible flow of energy between Larry and the trunk with its implements, and a tangible flow between me and the key which I sought to override with other flows of relationality.

The prison was also a lively presence on that morning. It was not just a place "in Larry's mind" that he was afraid of going back to, or a place that had caused him damage in the past, though it was still both of those things. His release from prison had been conditional on maintaining a record of good behaviour. He was "free", but the prison was ontologically and epistemologically present. For Larry, it was the plane of consisting in relation to which all meaning was made.

Our domestic life was shaped around prison-style routines. Breakfast, the same breakfast, would be served at the same hour, to the minute, every week-day. A packed lunch would be provided beside his porridge bowl, along with his freshly squeezed orange juice. This would all have been prepared while he shaved and showered. He would work all day at the university at his job as computer programmer, a job the prison authorities had secured for him, and return at 5.30, when his dinner would be served. After dinner he would water his vegetable garden, then return to his desk in the living room where he worked toward the completion of his maths honours degree. At that point the three small children must be kept silent. Not even a footfall could be allowed to disturb him. If the house was cold, he would wrap himself in a blanket. He did not allow us the luxury of heaters, though we lived in a very cold place.

The repetitive refrains that shaped the day could not be altered. There were to be no deviations. But cracks had begun to occur. There was a teacher shortage at the time, and I had been offered a teaching job – which I took. He tried to get me fired by lying to the Headmistress, but she had not taken the bait, telling me that other teachers' husbands had done the same thing. He got rid of the baby-sitter by terrifying her, but I found another. He went looking for another lover, but the women he approached were terrified of him. He needed a woman with guts he told me.

The strict routines of his prison were starting to fail him. But the prison had marked his body and that marked body made the chances of escape negligible. He had clumsy tattoos that had been made on his arms by other prisoners, that were evidently, to anyone who knew, prison tattoos. They had been necessary as proof to the other inmates that he was tough, an insider, despite the fact he spent all his hours in his cell studying. The Professor they called him. And he had missing teeth; prison dentistry consisted solely of pulling teeth out. He wore long sleeved shirts even in summer to cover his tattoos, and he had just had his remaining top teeth pulled out – all at once – and replaced with dentures so the gaps were no longer visible.

He wrote to the prison authorities to ask them to remove his record from the files so he could apply for a job elsewhere and escape the prison of his current life. They refused, writing to him that he would have to learn to live with his history. He did not believe he would be able to get a job elsewhere as his seven years in prison made too big a gap in his work record.

Then I escaped for a weekend with the children, and the unchanging system he had set up to enable him to endure, failed. He was profoundly shocked and exhausted. His trembling hands had fumbled his dentures and they had dropped and broken. When I returned and told him I would stay (the minister of my sister's church whom she had taken me to see, told me that, according to the Bible, women could only leave their husbands if their husbands ordered them to leave, and furthermore, he said, our deaths would not be a problem if he killed us, as it would be God's will). Clinging on to the thin straw of another assemblage, I told Larry I would stay. But it was too late. He no longer had a life that could endure, and a week later he was dead.

What was it to be Larry, struggling to endure, and failing? This is not solely a story of gendered violence. It is also a story of the violence done to young men and boys when they are incarcerated – a violence they might never find the way to uncouple themselves from. It is about the way small, seemingly insignificant things, a tattoo, a possum, a stuck lock, a key hidden in a packet of Bex up high at the back of the laundry cupboard, among other things, intra-acted to create the assemblage through which a marriage and a life ended. It is about the response-ability of those things, animate, and apparently inanimate, generating patterns of human life and death. It is about the deadening effect of lines of descent that have lost the way to respond to lines of ascent. It is about time that is not linear and events that never end. "A scar is the sign not of a past wound but of 'the present fact of having been wounded': we can say that it is the contemplation of the wound, that it contracts all the instants which separate us from it into a living present" (Deleuze, 2004: 98–99).

And so...

This turn to agential matter/ing has required a radical re-thinking of the relationship between the human and the more-than-human world. In this turn, it is argued that more-than-human others, including photos and works of art, are not inert, passive objects in the service, beautification and edification of humanity. They are not seen as discrete objects, but the lively "stuff" of matter that is articulate and agential: "feeling, desiring and experiencing are not singular characteristics or capacities of human consciousness. Matter feels, converses, suffers, desires, yearns and remembers" (Barad, 2011: 59).

References

Barad, K. 2007. *Meeting the Universe Halfway*. Durham, NC/London: Duke University Press.

Barad, K. 2010. Quantum entanglements and hauntological relations of inheritance: Dis/continuities, spacetime enfoldings, and justice-to-come. *Derrida Today*, 3(2), 240–268.

Barad, K. 2011. Interview with Karen Barad. In R. Dolphijn and I. van der Tuin (eds), *New Materialism: Interviews and Cartographies*. Ann Arbor, MI: Open Humanities Press, 48–70.

Barad, K. 2015. On touching the inhuman that therefore I am (vol. 1). In K. Stakemeier and S. Witzgall (eds), *Power of Material/Politics of Materiality*. Zurich, SW: Diaphanes, 153–164.

Bennett, J. 2010. *Vibrant matter. A Political Ecology of Things*. Durham, NC: Duke University Press.

Bennett, J. 2012. Powers of the hoard: Further notes on material agency. In J. J. Cohen (ed.), *Animal, Vegetable, Mineral: Ethics and Objects*. Washington, DC: Oliphaunt Books, Punctum Press, 237–272.

Bergson, H. 1998. *Creative Evolution* (trans. A. Mitchell). Mineola, NY: Dover Publications Inc.

Blackman, L. 2015. Researching affect and embodied hauntologies: Exploring an analytics of experimentation. In B. T. Knudsen and C. Stage (eds), *Affective Methodologies: Developing Cultural Research Strategies for the Study of Affect*. London: Palgrave Macmillan, 25–44.

Bright, D. 2018. Signs to be developed: Experiments in writing. In S. Riddle, D. Bright and E. Honan (eds), *Writing with Deleuze in the Academy: Creating Monsters*. Singapore: Springer, 95–105.

Davies, B. 2018. The persistent smile of the Cheshire Cat. Explorations in the agency of matter through art-making. *Qualitative Inquiry*, 1–9. DOI: 10.1177/1077800418809742.

de Freitas, E. 2017. Karen Barad's quantum ontology and posthuman ethics. Rethinking the concept of relationality. *Qualitative Inquiry*, 23(9), 741–748.

Deleuze, G. 1980. *Cours Vincennes 12/21/1980*. http://www.webdeleuze.com/php/texte.php?cle=190andgroupe=Spinoza andlangue=2) (accessed 10 February 2010).

Deleuze, G. 2004. *Difference and Repetition* (trans. P. Patton). London: Continuum.

Deleuze, G. 2005. *Pure Immanence. Essays on a Life*. New York: Zone Books

Deleuze, G. and Guattari, F. 1987. *A Thousand Plateaus: Capitalism and Schizophrenia* (trans. B. Massumi). Minneapolis, MN: University of Minnesota Press.

Grosz, E. 2008. *Chaos, Territory, Art: Deleuze and the Framing of the Earth*. New York: Columbia University Press.

Hill, J. 2019. *See What You Made Me Do. Power, control and domestic abuse*. Carlton, Vic: Black Inc.

Thomson, J., Linnell, S., Laws, C. and Davies, B. 2018. Entanglements between art-making and storytelling in a collective biography on the death of an intimate other. *Departures in Critical Qualitative Inquiry*, 7(3), 4–26.

Wyatt, J., Gale, K., Gannon, S. and Davies, B. 2011. *Deleuze and Collaborative Writing: An Immanent Plane of Composition*. New York: Peter Lang.

5

COLLECTIVE BIOGRAPHY

A diffractive methodology

> In which I explore collective biography as a diffractive methodology. I explore the materiality of words and stories and work with a memory from a collective biography workshop on the topic of death of an intimate other. The memory and the artwork, which lie at the heart of this chapter, were emergent in intra-action with the collective biography participants in that workshop, along with their stories, their artwork and the place we worked in. The memory I work with takes up the story of the end of my marriage, as told in Chapter 4.

In Chapter 4, I explored the power of things in terms of response-ability, coming into being in always emergent entanglements with others whom they affect and are affected by. I re-visited a workshop in which the participants learned to read others from invisible energy fields, including those emanating from things they had held for some time in their possession. And then I returned to the assemblage of the end of my marriage, and worked toward a different reading of it, a different sense of it, by focusing on the agency of the apparently inanimate things that were entangled in that assemblage. I turn again, here, in this chapter, to that event, through the collective biography on the death of an intimate other (Thomson et al., 2018). Through returning, again, I explore the diffractive methodology of collective biography.

The method of collective biography was originally inspired by the memory-work of Frigga Haug and her collective in *Female Sexualization: A Collective Work of Memory* (1987). The Haug collective worked with early memories of their bodies, with the intention of making women's lives and bodies relevant in Marxist theory, which was dominant at that time. It wasn't just Marxist theory that was gender blind in the 1980s; social constructionism, similarly, situated itself in men's lives, and favoured mind and rationality over embodiment and emotion (Davies, 1987).

Collective biography began in the 1990s, inspired by such work, and by feminist theorising taking place in a range of disciplines, including human, literary and biological sciences, which were contributing to the deconstruction of the male/female and mind/body binaries. In the early days of collective biography we drew our concepts primarily from Butler and Foucault; later we turned to Deleuze and to Barad (Davies and Gannon, 2006, 2009, 2013). In this chapter I draw again on the concept of diffraction in order to examine what it is that collective biography can do:

> Diffraction marks the limits of the determinacy and permanency of boundaries. One of the crucial lessons we learn is that agential cuts cut things together and apart. Diffraction is a matter of differential entanglements; this is the deep significance of a diffraction pattern .
>
> (Barad, 2008: 333)

In collective biography workshops, which usually extend over several days, the participants work with their memories to explore the intra-active becoming of entangled subjects. The purpose of the memory-work is not to reveal or represent individualised identities, but to explore the impersonal, immanent singularities that are emergent in the memories our research topics give rise to. And its purpose is not to elaborate difference and injustice, in terms of categories of difference, but to explore the processes of differenciation, that is, the ongoing process of becoming. Through the memory work of the participants it explores the specificity or singularity of becoming. While it is cognisant of the strata and of the processes of territorialisation that lock some into powerful positions while depriving others of power, its focus is on the moment-by-moment immanence of lives, and as Coleman and Ringrose (2013: 10) point out: "Immanence refers to the specificity or singularity of a thing; not to what can be made to fit into a pre-existent abstraction."

The work of producing those singular memories in collective biography workshops is simultaneously physical, linguistic and intra-active. It is physical in so far as telling stories and later reading them out loud involves the vibrating bodies of both teller and listeners. It is linguistic in so far as the storytellers are attentive to the language they use, avoiding clichés, explanations and moral judgements. Participants tell their memory stories as much as possible from the embodied detail of the experiences of the participants in their remembered story. And it is intra-active, in so far as the listeners work with each storyteller, as their stories are unfolded into the space of the workshop, listening with sympathy, in such a way that they come to know the experience from inside itself. At the same time, they listen with ears pricked for clichés and explanations or moral judgements that might get in the way of the story's fleshiness. It is physical, too, when it comes to writing the stories, when each participant is involved in mark-making on the page or screen, and sometimes too in image making or other forms of artmaking. The process of writing and of artmaking involves each participant in sympoiesis – a collective knowing in being. The mark-making and mark-shaping tools are also active participants in the process of memory work, as are the artworks they generate, and the poems and stories that are written. Further, the concepts the participants work with are both epistemologically and ontologically alive – they are no longer abstract, but rather are written down, talked about and put to work in relation to the stories as they and the participants explore what work they are capable of – what knowing in being they can intra-actively give rise to. Memory stories are told, written, read out loud, listened to, discussed, re-written; and in that process they eliminate disembodied clichés, facile explanations and moral judgements. They move from the singular to the collective. They are lively and responsive.

Before turning to the workshop on the death of an intimate other, I want to pause, and focus on that liveliness and responsiveness of memories. To do that, I turn to a story told in a chapter that I wrote about my father, Tom, in *New Lives in an Old Land* (Davies, 2019a). Through that story I make the emergent entanglement of memory visible and tangible.

The liveliness of words

I wrote about my father's fear of heights:

> As I think about my father, all these years later, I remember a man who was tightly controlled and afraid of chaos – of falling or drowning. When we drove over the mountains to the beach, we (that is, we kids and our Mum) loved to stop and look at Ebor Falls, the highest waterfall in the state, but Tom couldn't bear to go anywhere near it. Seeing us look over the waterfall made him sick.
>
> (Davies, 2019a: 84)

The trouble is, I discovered, after the book was published, that Ebor Falls is not the highest falls in the state. When one of my readers pointed that out to me, I was mortified. I *knew* they weren't the highest falls in the state, yet through multiple drafts of the chapter I had not corrected that error. I hadn't even noticed it.

Blackman writes about the liveliness of the words we utter, and of their capacity, "to *perform* a series of displaced, submerged, disqualified, or disavowed relations that might undo the present and open to lost futures" (Blackman, 2015: 28; emphasis added). And Haraway points out that words have a different liveliness once the epistemology/ontology binary is rejected. She refers to sentences as organisms (Haraway, 2018). And indeed it seemed as if those words, "the highest waterfall in the state", had taken on a particular liveliness that was capable of evading my careful editing. The story I told, far from transparently recording or representing my father's identity, was itself an event in the ongoing multiplicity of our entangled lives.

So what were some of the entanglements in this slippage of mine? My father was very much given to hyperbole. He loved to tell us our house was the best in the town, the climate of our town was the best in the world, his sons would be prime ministers. In animating my father in writing about him, and in writing of his fear of heights, I cut together his love of hyperbole with his fear of heights. This was not an intentional cut. If we think of words as lively then at least some of the agency in that cut might be said to belong to the words.

Rather than being the agent in control of my text, I was entangled, as I wrote that small story, in my father's fear, and in my own memory of the waterfall. The slippage into hyperbole, claiming the waterfall was the highest in the state, could work to make my father's fear appear to be quite reasonable.

In this diffractive cutting together-apart, time is indeterminate. "*For any given event, there is indeterminacy as to when it occurred or began or ended.* Temporality is itself indeterminate" (de Freitas, 2017: 743). My father is long gone but his verbal strategies are still lively. His fear of that waterfall is as lively now as it was then. We know lives, Barad points out, through "the pattern of sedimented enfoldings of iterative intra-activity – [which] is written into the fabric of the world" (Barad, 2010: 261).

And as Atwood (1988: 3) says: "You don't look back along time but down through it, like water. Sometimes this comes to the surface, sometimes that, sometimes nothing. Nothing goes away". "The world 'holds' the memory of all traces; or rather the world is its memory (enfolded materialisation)" (Barad, 2010: 261). The world in all its iterative intra-activity holds that memory of my father. Discovering that cut, that slippage, was provoking. I worried about the apparent unreliability of my memory, and about my apparent untrustworthiness as one who traces the details of the events she has been entangled in. So I decided to revisit the waterfall, this time writing not to tell a story about anyone, as if anyone is ever one and not many, but to allow the event of visiting the waterfall to rise to the surface, as I have learned to do in collective biography workshops.

> We were on our way from our home on the Liverpool Plains to our summer holiday at the beach. It was a long, seven-hour journey up over the Great Dividing Range. The tiny, misty village of Ebor was the highest point on our journey.
>
> It had been raining a lot lately and Mum wanted to see the water flowing over the Falls. Dad never liked to stop anywhere, especially at the Falls, but we joined Mum in pestering him, and so he pulled off the road and drove to the head of the Falls. From the carpark to the edge of the Falls was bright green grass and smooth stretches of granite filled with the roaring sound of the water. I climbed gingerly out of the car, where I had been squashed for queasy hours with my three siblings, breathing the thick, sick-making smoke of my parents' cigarettes.
>
> Tony's body exploded into action, car door wide open, running toward the Falls. The others followed more slowly. My father stood still by the car, his hand on the bonnet, as if he had lost his balance. He called out to us, in a tight voice, not to go too close. The air was icy and fresh. My trembling legs moved forward to join the others. How close do I have to go to that edge in order not to draw attention to my fear?

I found this wonderful photo of Ebor Falls in flood on a Google website. The other photos on the site are beautiful, but clichéd and predictable – they could be waterfalls anywhere with their picture-perfect cascading, multi-level falls. This photo is different, holding all the surging power of the water, alive with the force of the potential energy of the drop.

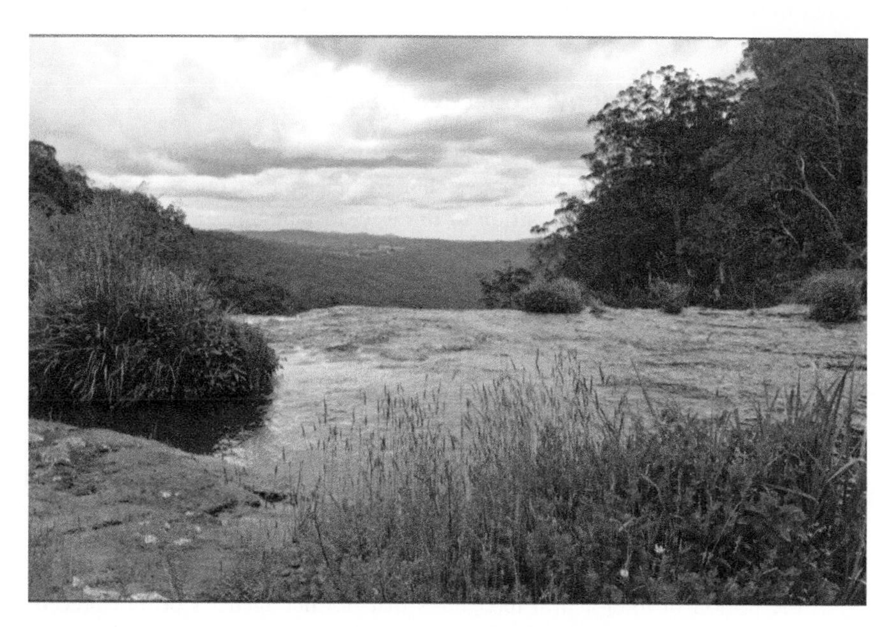

FIGURE 5.1 Ebor Falls in flood. Photograph by Belinda Turner. Google Knowledge Panel on the Google site for Ebor Falls, 2020.

The event of visiting Ebor Falls is tucked into the folds and interstices of the world that also hold my father, his fear *and my own*, and the means of disguising that fear with hyperbole – his own as well as mine. The world holds, too, the ice-cold air, the mist, the frozen fingers and noses, and my stiff, car-sick body – and the exhilaration of the water tumbling down over the vertical rock face, the fine mist spray rising high in the cold mountain air.

In allowing the event to expand, a simple small story that relied on an untruth for its purchase, the child and the father come alive along with the fear of the fall; the entanglement between me and my father rises to the surface, it re-emerges, and at the same time its liveliness means it goes on multiplying and differenciating itself.

Let me return, then, with this understanding of the liveliness of words to collective biography as a diffractive methodology, where the human participants respond to each other's memories, where time is no longer linear – where past becomes present and unfolds into different possible futures, futures already affecting the past and the present. Diffraction is like two waves meeting in the ocean, responding to each other, changing the shape and direction of each other; but it is not just about these large forces intra-acting. Each wave is more than itself, intra-acting with forces larger than itself, the moon, the sun, the body of the ocean, the seasons, the surface of the ocean floor, and a multitude of smaller forces inside-outside itself such that there can be no clear demarcation between wave and not-wave.

Diffractive methodology: Collective biography

A diffractive methodology takes into account the multiplicative lines of force at work with/in the events that the researcher-participants set out to explore. The concept of diffraction draws attention to the ways in which participants affect and are affected by lines of force; lines of force that are ethical, ontological, and epistemological. The research inquiry is itself a line of force. It makes things happen. It is *intra-active*. In the work of collective biography, the researcher-participants are open to being surprised, and being affected, by the concepts, by their encounters, by the material they produce and are produced by, and by their talking, writing, reading out loud, and by their intra-active, emergent listening.

What emerges in the event of a collective biography is not a record of what existed before the event; it is not a study of pre-existing entities and identities, but of intra-active relationality as it emerges:

> the notion of intra-action recognizes that distinct agencies do not precede, but rather emerge through, their intra-action. It is important to note that 'distinct' agencies are only distinct in a relational, not an absolute, sense, that is, agencies are only distinct in relation to their mutual entanglement; they don't exist as individual elements. Crucially, the notion of intra-action constitutes *a radical reworking of the traditional notion of causality*.
>
> (Barad, 2008: 325 fn14; emphasis added)

The participant-researchers in a collective biography, usually a small group of four to six people, do not just tell ready-made stories – they enter into an intra-active relationality; they affect each other. They are affected physically, emotionally — in their knowing-in-being — in their becoming. They are only distinct in "their mutual entanglement". In each workshop the process is emergent, though there are also methodic practices that are followed. In one workshop, for example, in which we set out to research the topic of embodied women at work in neoliberal institutions (Davies et al., 2006), we followed the process of telling, listening, writing, reading out loud, open discussion, rewriting and reading again out loud. We cooked together, ate together and walked together. In telling stories we also often laughed and cried together. We were also inventive in different ways suited to the topic in hand. For example, we developed strategies to remind us to pay attention to our bodies:

> These included a guided yoga nidra, voice work, foot massage, and a guided visualization. While these strategies were initially conceived of as a way to take care of our bodies alongside our academic work, they also provided a way to keep the body in central focus *in* our academic work.
>
> (Davies et al., 2006: 66)

The work of collective biography depends on the response-ability of the researcher-participants. They respond to each other, and to the participants within the memory stories that they tell, and they respond to the stories themselves, along with works of art, when they are produced, and to the physical setting in which the memories are told. The workshop is itself a diffractive assemblage with immediately evident forces (the wave-like human participants) intra-acting, emerging, differenciating, and the multiplicative, less evident forces, exerting their thing-power, making their presence felt.

Ideally, the workshop venue is free of the demands and stresses of everyday neoliberal, institutional life. Two collective biographies I have run, which failed to generate anything new, were conducted in university offices and meeting rooms. Such spaces demand attention, and participants have trouble letting go of the relations of power and of the values that attach to their institutional positions. Securing funding to escape the forces at play in such settings can sometimes run into trenchant opposition – as it did in those two failed workshops. One Dean asserted that our research grant could not be spent on a house that could be described as beautiful or pleasurable. When I asked him what would count as sufficiently ugly, he was at something of a loss, though he did suggest it might mean nowhere near the ocean. He was worried that we might be seen to be enjoying ourselves – neoliberalism is captured by appearances. Luckily the funding rules were against him, and we were able to rent the house by the sea where we put together the first draft of the book *Pedagogical Encounters* (Davies and Gannon, 2009).

It is vital that participants in collective biographies are free to bring total attention to their virtual, immanent embodiment, when they return to the experiences in their memory stories, and as they experience the telling/writing/reading/listening in the participatory event of the workshop. Some ideal locations have been Magnetic Island, off the North Queensland coast, where we rented a house in a tropical paradise across the road from the ocean; another was in Bombo, south of Sydney in New South Wales, in a house with wide views out over the Pacific Ocean where whales spouted and cavorted while we worked on our stories sitting around a log fire; and yet another was a cosy house in the Belgian countryside where we could sit in the sunshine around a large wooden table in a lush, flowering garden. In each of these houses, and in many others, the co-researchers have lived, cooked and eaten together, spending the day talking, listening, writing, reading-out-loud, crying, laughing, rewriting, artmaking, talking some more, then planning the paper they will subsequently write after going back to their everyday lives.

Reflection and reflexivity have been so taken-for-granted in conceptualising what we do in qualitative research, that diffraction as metaphor and practice makes for an interesting shift in our thinking about what we do and the cuts we make. Reflection and reflexivity maintain the primacy of the individual who reflects, and they assume a reality that exists independent of the act of reflection. Their tendency is to deploy categories of difference, such as gender, class, sexuality, ethnicity, (dis)ability, for example, into which we can each be sorted, and through which we can each be explained. In a diffractive analysis those categories explain nothing and are themselves in need of explanation. Diffraction is interested in, and itself implicated in, the process whereby a *difference is made*. What a diffractive methodology sets out to do is to track the interference patterns, and to discover from them the ongoing processes through which the world creates, and goes on creating, itself. A diffractive approach opens up, within the research, an ethico-onto-epistemological space of *emergent encounter*. The diffractive researcher's task is not to tell of something or someone that exists independent of, or prior to, the research encounter, but to access that which is becoming true in the moment of encounter. In telling, writing, reading, listening to and rewriting our memory stories in collective biography workshops, we are *not only* accessing what was once true, but opening up a space in which some thing new can emerge. A diffractive research encounter is in this sense experimental; researchers in a collective biography workshop do not know in advance what knowledge will emerge, or how that knowledge will matter.

The nature of the listening and responding in collective biography is the key. Each participant, in listening to the others, seeks to know, in listening, and questioning, what it was and is to be in those moments of the others' memory stories. In collectively coming to know each moment – each diffractive mo(ve)ment – as it is re-lived in the telling and writing and reading out loud to each other, the participants contribute to the emergence of each other's stories, and they come to know their own stories differently. It is a process of emergent listening (Davies, 2014, 2016).

The questioning of my initial story of my father took place not in a workshop, but came from a reader. The discovery of the error gave rise to a burst of energy and to a rewriting of the event at the Falls. Emergent listening moves beyond moral judgement (in this case the judgement that I was not a reliable story-teller) towards recognition of the other, and towards an affective openness to emergent entangled differences.

Openness to encounters with the other, to being affected by the other, is not just to encounters with other humans, but also to the material world in all its manifestations – a material-social-epistemological world that one is emergent *with*. To engage with others, diffractively, in this way means that the research event is ethical, *and* open *and* evolving. As Barad says of ethics, it is

> about responsibility and accountability for the lively relationalities of becoming, of which we are a part. Ethics is about mattering, about taking account of

> the entangled materializations of which we are part, including new configurations, new subjectivities, new possibilities. Even the smallest cuts matter. Responsibility is then a matter of the ability to respond. *Listening for the response of the other and an obligation to be responsive to the other, who is not entirely separate from what we call the self.*
>
> (Barad, 2011: 69; emphasis added)

Emergent listening in collective biography workshops *intra-acts with the mode of telling* – a deliberate cutting away of clichés, explanations and moral judgements, telling and listening and retelling from particular bodies, in emergent relations with other bodies, human and more-than-human. The participants write and engage in artmaking, not to reveal (or discover) an essential self that existed in the past, but to bring both self and other into the moment and movement, and into the immanent, diffractive becoming, where present, past and future dissolve into the *spacetime* of working together.

Contrary to research practice that attempts to re-present pre-existing entities, collective biography works in the mo(ve)ment that is created among the participants during the workshop, and in the analysis and writing after the workshop. It is, in Deleuze and Guattari's (1994) terms, ambulatory; lines of descent are necessary to give shape and form, and sometimes permission, to the research, but sometimes they need to be erased in order to give way to lines of ascent.

In writing from the body, rather than relying on well-worn clichés, explanations and moral judgements, collective biography lets in that breath of fresh air from the chaos.

In the early days of collective biographies (for example, Davies et al., 2001) we would meet for a week in rented accommodation where we could live, eat and go for long walks together, and take time to talk about our other ongoing research projects. These days, given the increased time pressure from the neoliberalised institutions in which we work (Brown, 2003), two days tends to be the maximum time that participants can afford to be away from their 'work'; occasionally we manage to negotiate three.

The methodic practices of collective biography evolve; they respond creatively to the time and place, the participants, and the particular research question they have decided to pursue. The method emerges, through the work done together, as a research assemblage:

> Assemblages are not simply objects or things, but qualities, speeds, flows and lines of force. Their character is defined not by what they are, but by what they can do, or become. And they are always in the process of becoming, not through an intention to arrive at a pre-determined end-point, but through multiple encounters with emergent multiplicities.
>
> (Bansel and Davies, 2014: 41)

In this sense, the talking, writing and artmaking in collective biography is a performative practice of the not-yet-thought, or to put it another way, the "nonthought within thought" (Deleuze and Guattari, 1994: 51). Our "non-thought" creatively evolves through our memory stories and our artmaking, putting imagination to work in intra-action with conceptual analysis. We seek, in Bennett's (2010: 14) words, "a shared, vital materiality" or collective, embodied liveliness.

The death of an intimate other

I turn now to the recent collective biography I participated in with a group of colleagues on the topic of the death of an intimate other (Thomson et al., 2018). The workshop was inspired by Thomson's research with art therapists working with people who are dying (Thomson, 2019a, 2019b). In that workshop we planned from the outset to include artmaking alongside our story telling/writing/reading/listening. While artmaking is not always practiced in collective biography workshops, in this workshop it was a particular focus of our work. Thomson's previous interviews with art therapists had used artmaking as an integral part of her interviews, and she was planning to use artmaking in her collective biographies with art therapists. Our work together was a methodological experiment, developed in anticipation of the workshops she would run with art therapists.

Our workshop took place over two consecutive days in the art therapy teaching studio at Western Sydney University. This was a vast, new, purpose-built room with steel benches running down the middle, and small rooms to retreat into off to the side. Along one wall were sliding glass doors looking out on to a sheltered outdoor space, and beyond that abundant green grass. Just inside the glass doors were some beautiful, old art-therapy tables, spattered and soaked with paint and scratches, mellowed and worn with sweat and tears. We gravitated to those old tables. So yes, we were in an institution that reeked of royal-legal practices and products, and that carried a certain risk of de-railing us. But we were also in a space that was new enough not to have absorbed the oppressive affects of neoliberalism with its relentless lines of descent (Davies, 2019b). The history of art-therapy teaching in this particular university was one of successfully managing those lines of descent, and at the same time bypassing them. The old tables carried the history of students' lines of flight in their artwork, and gave us permission to amble off whatever path the institution might have imagined we were on.

We began our two days together with coffee and relaxed getting-to-know-each-other talk, before settling around the big table by the windows to begin our story telling. We listened closely to each other's stories, asking for clarification when we didn't understand them – or couldn't imagine our way into them. The processes of telling, listening, retelling, questioning, lapped seamlessly over each other. After we finished our story telling we separated into different parts of the studio to write our stories, seeking places of solitude and quiet contemplation that would enable the embodied details of our stories to find their way on to page or screen.

The challenge of telling, writing and making art in relation to a memory, without resorting to cliché, explanation or moral judgement is a major one. Participants often feel inadequate to the task, so embedded are their memories in those three features. However hard we work at it, those clichés, explanations and judgements inevitably find their way into our written stories. The listeners open themselves to being in the moment, to participating in the movement, of the story being told. At the same time, they take note of those clunky moments when clichés, explanations and moral judgements get in the way. They listen in such a way that they enable each storyteller to tell the story from inside itself, from inside the collective of research participants. It is in that collective vitality that mo(ve)ment takes place, from individual memory to collective emergence of a multiple, fluid vitality.

When we finished our story telling and writing we had lunch together at the outdoor café, allowing our minds to collectively wander over the many events that currently concerned us. We didn't talk about our morning's work, but in that relaxed time together, where talk wandered wherever it would, the artworks we were about to make were emergent in our bodies even while we paid no conscious attention to them.

After lunch, we moved to art making and then to writing about the art making itself. In both of these activities the memories took on a new form. Listening to the written stories read out loud and responding to the artworks brought more questions, as the participants worked once more to know the memory from inside itself in its emerging multiplicity and entangled lines of force.

In this particular workshop we discovered, to our surprise, that moral judgement of ourselves had seeped into our story telling, escaping our notice. We had each judged ourselves as somehow inadequate to the task we had faced. The stories we were telling were of events that had taken place decades earlier, in the 1960s, 1970s and 1980s. Each of us had written about someone with whom we had had a significant or intimate relationship. We were young women of about the same age then, young to be given responsibilities we were unprepared for. Our stories and our art works contained moments of power and of incapacity, of control and helplessness, of death and survival. My own story was of the death of my husband. It took place when I was 25 years old, though I felt at the time much, much older. My story, lodged in the fabric of the world, in the world that I am *of*, was as follows.

> He packed some underclothes into his briefcase, and into his shirt pocket he placed the sympathetic, concerned letter his mother had recently written to me, in response to my telling her about his increasing violence. Her letter had infuriated him, and as for me, I didn't have "the guts" he said, that he needed in a wife.
>
> Now he stood at the front door, flinging words back at me – words that I had spoken when he had returned earlier than usual from work. Everything had to stop when he walked in that door. The life and liveliness of my life with the children stopped. They could no longer play; they must remain silent so as not to bother him. The house must be immaculately clean and tidy, all

toys packed away. His dinner must be on the table by the time he finished watering the vegetable garden. When he had walked in early that day, the words "It's like black death when you walk in that door" had sprung out of my mouth, unbidden. Now he repeated them back to me, adding "You'll never see me again", leaving me in no doubt his death was to be my responsibility. The letter in his pocket would let his mother know she too must share the blame; she had betrayed him by writing to me in sympathy.

He drove into town to the insurance office where he cancelled his life insurance policy, to the bank where he took what money he had out of his account and sent it to his father. He bought a bicycle tube, and then he drove to Sydney.

I rang his mother and told her I could do no more. I was exhausted. I had nothing left to give him, I said. I could take care of him no longer. I told her he was on his way to Goulburn, where he would attempt to kill two screws he still hated. He would then kill himself. It was a well-rehearsed story. The alternative had been that he would kill all of us, but that one was no longer the story that was playing itself out.

She didn't believe me. She said he'd be back. I was over-reacting. She didn't see any need to do anything. I told her again I could do no more; I was handing her the chance to intervene if she wished. Poor woman, she would never forgive herself for not taking me seriously.

He stayed overnight in Sydney with his aunt, who didn't guess anything was wrong. He drove to Goulburn next day. He didn't kill anyone, but he did kill himself, with my sleeping pills, pills prescribed because of my night terrors, in which I became a small thin scream falling in a bottomless chasm, confiscated because it was unthinkable that I might sleep so soundly that I would fail to get up to the babies when they cried. With the confiscated sleeping pills and the bicycle tube stretched from the exhaust to the hatchback door, on a lonely dirt road, he died as day sank into night, the bright interior of the car lit up like a candle flame in the dark night.

Late that night two policemen came to my door to tell me he was dead. I hadn't been able to sleep. I had been waiting for them. I asked if anyone else had died in Goulburn that day and they told me no. "Thank god for that," I said. I didn't ask them in, and nor did they ask to come in like they do in the soaps. I was 25 years old. The children were four, two and one.

My brother, newly graduated from law school, sat up with me all night, pondering the question of whether I was guilty. The prison system had handed him into my care. It had been my job to support him as he made his way back into life on the "outside". I had failed the task they had given me. My brother questioned me on all I had done and all I might have done if I could have found the right person to help, and at the end of the night he decided I was not guilty. An incredible gift, though the words I'd spoken weighed on me heavily.

When we came back from lunch I sat down at the old wooden table and drew the image that had been growing not just over lunch, but that I had been awake most of the night before thinking about. I had in the past written of my marriage being like a rock that my life, like the roots of a tree, must grow around (Wyatt and Davies, 2011). On my daily walk, there are Moreton Bay Fig trees with enormous roots that visibly wind their way over and around rocks – even rock walls. I had taken photos of some of those trees to help me draw the roots of my tree – my life – growing around that rock.

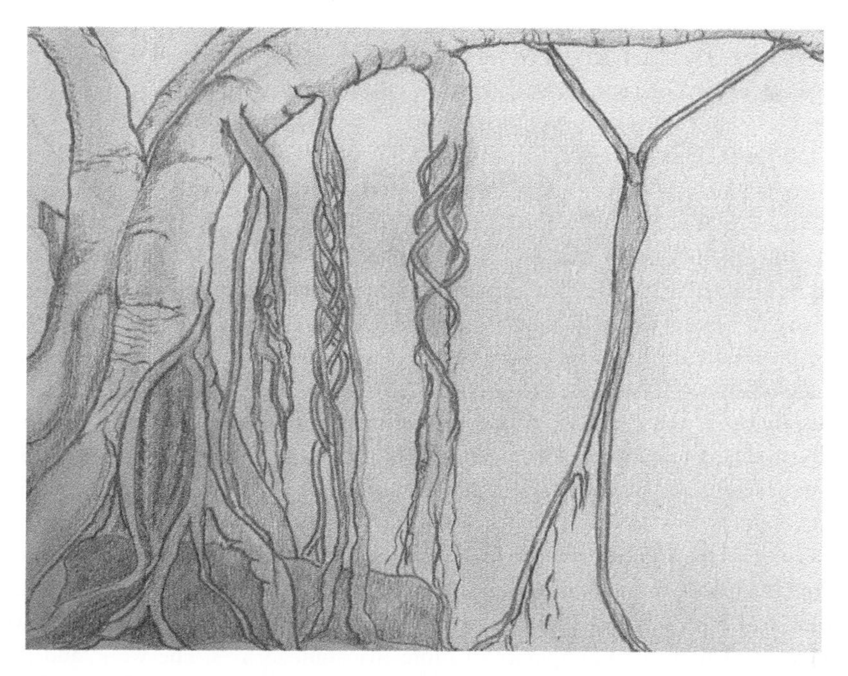

FIGURE 5.2 Bronwyn Davies, Moreton Bay fig.
2018, detail. Photograph by Bronwyn Davies, 2020.

The tree in my drawing rises up on the left margin of the page and reaches out across the top. It's another version of the tree I have drawn again and again when doodling on the margins of papers at endless boring meetings. This tree seems different – it is more fluid, more muscular, and it has found a way to support itself with aerial roots that could potentially turn it from tree into forest.

At the time I drew it in the workshop the hard, relentless work of the roots in holding up the branch, in supporting the trunk, the life, *a* life, that will go on growing in spite of the rock, and the huge wound in the trunk, brought tears to my eyes. The trunk and the main branch are strong and solid, vital and fleshy, while the aerial roots are more tentative, perhaps even fragile. I thought at the time, it's just a pencil drawing. I could rub it all out. But I didn't, of course. The image I had created on the page affected me, it held me. It had taken on its own force. I had planned to trace over the pencil lines with ink, but their transience seemed integral to the artwork, however disturbing I might find that thought.

One of the significant movements in-between our storying and artmaking was the realisation that we had all judged ourselves and found ourselves lacking. We had all spoken and written of ourselves as inadequate and helpless in the face of death. We were four strong, competent, feminist women, yet, in telling our stories about the ways in which we had faced the death of an intimate other, we had judged ourselves harshly. Our stories, in spite of the injunction not to engage in moral judgement, had made a judgement of weakness and incompetence that we were barely aware of at the time, and we had done so, in spite of the considerable presence of elements in our stories that told otherwise.

Our artmaking made visible and palpable the weight of the forces that had demanded more of us than we could bear – and yet, what we struggled to recognise was that not only had we borne them, but that we had done so with extraordinary strength and a resilience that we might celebrate. In my case the vulnerability that had crept into my story had, in a peculiar way, protected me from blame. It was as if the line of descent that told of victimhood and weakness was a "roll ready prepared" that in principle "might be accomplished almost instantaneously, like releasing a spring" (Bergson, 1998: 11).

Looking at the drawing, now, two years later, I am startled at how strong the trunk and branch are. The rock has become inconsequential, and the aerial roots are light and playful. I am deeply moved by its strength and vitality, and its mo(ve)ment.

Our storying and our artwork involved us in intra-active becoming as entangled subjects. Our work focused not on identities, but on the intra-active singularities of life, and of death. Our strategies were both systematic and ambulatory; and we had worked with the multiplicity of more-than-human lives. The work, and the subsequent writing and thinking called on rationality, sensation and affect, working with the movement between participants, not just the flesh-and-blood participants, but also the ghost participants and the more-than-human participants of our stories, scrubbing away some of the old clichés, opening up spaces for lines of ascent through which, in this case, old stories of women being inadequate, or guilty, could be given the flick – at least for now.

References

Atwood, M. 1988. *Cat's Eye*. New York: Doubleday.

Bansel, P. and Davies, B. 2014. Assembling Oscar, assembling South Africa, assembling affects. *Emotion Space & Society*, 13, 40–45. doi:10.1016/j.emospa.2014.04.002.

Barad, K. 2008. Queer causation and the ethics of mattering. In M. J. Hyrd and N. Giffney (eds), *Queering the Non/Human*. Taylor & Francis Group. ProQuest Ebook, 247–352.

Barad, K. 2010. Quantum entanglements and hauntological relations of inheritance: Dis/continuities, spacetime enfoldings, and justice-to-come. *Derrida Today*, 3(2), 240–268.

Barad, K. 2011. Interview with Karen Barad. In R. Dolphijn and I. van der Tuin (eds.), *New Materialism: Interviews and Cartographies*. Ann Arbor, MI: Open Humanities Press, 48–70.

Bennett, J. 2010. *Vibrant matter: A Political Ecology of Things*. Durham, NC: Duke University Press.

Bergson, H. 1998. *Creative Evolution* (trans. A. Mitchell). Mineola, NY: Dover Publications Inc.

Blackman, L. 2015. Researching affect and embodied hauntologies: exploring an analytics of experimentation. In B.T. Knudsen and C. Stage (eds). *Affective Methodologies: Developing Cultural Research Strategies for the Study of Affect*. London UK: Palgrave Macmillan.

Brown, W. 2003. Neo-liberalism and the end of liberal democracy. *Theory and Event*, 7(1), 1–43.

Coleman, R. and Ringrose, J. 2013. Introduction. In R. Coleman and J. Ringrose (eds), *Deleuze and Research Methodologies*. Edinburgh: Edinburgh University Press, 1–22.

Davies, B. 1987. Marriage and the construction of reality revisited: An exercise in rewriting social theory to include women's experience. *Educational Philosophy and Theory*, 19 (1), 20–28.

Davies, B. 2014. *Listening to Children: Being and Becoming*. London: Routledge.

Davies, B. 2016. Emergent listening. In N. K. Denzin and M. D. Giardina (eds), *Qualitative Inquiry through a Critical Lens*. New York: Routledge, 73–84.

Davies, B. 2019a. *New Lives in an Old Land: Re-turning to the Colonization of New South Wales through Stories of my Parents and their Ancestors*. Sydney, NSW: Ornythorhynchus Paradoxus Books.

Davies, B. 2019b. Life in neoliberal institutions: Australian stories. *Qualitative Inquiry*, 1–7. DOI: 10.1177/10778004|9878737.

Davies, B. and Gannon, S. (eds) 2006. *Doing Collective Biography*. Maidenhead, UK: Open University Press.

Davies, B. and Gannon, S. (eds) 2009. *Pedagogical Encounters*. New York: Peter Lang.

Davies, B. and Gannon, S. 2013. Collective biography and the entangled enlivening of being. *International Review of Qualitative Research*, 5(4), 357–376.

Davies, B., Dormer, S., Gannon, S., Laws, C., Lenz-Taguchi, H., McCann, H. and Rocco, S. 2001. Becoming schoolgirls: The ambivalent project of subjectification. *Gender and Education*, 13(2), 167–182.

Davies, B., Browne, J., Gannon, S., Honan, E. and Somerville, M. 2006. Embodied women at work in neoliberal times and places. In Davies, B. and Gannon, S. (eds), *Doing Collective Biography*. Maidenhead, UK: Open University Press, 61–78.

de Freitas, E. 2017. Karen Barad's quantum ontology and posthuman ethics. Rethinking the concept of relationality. *Qualitative Inquiry*, 23(9), 741–748.

Deleuze, G. and Guattari, F. 1994. *What Is Philosophy?* (trans. H. Tomlinson and G. Burchell). New York: Columbia University Press.

Haraway, D. 2018 1997). (*Modest_Witness@Second_Millennium: Female_Man©_Meets_OncomouseTM* 2nd Edition. New York and London: Routledge.

Haug, F. 1987. *Female Sexualization: A Collective Work of Memory* (trans. E. Carter). London: Verso Press.

Thomson, J. 2019a. The work of art therapy: An immersive visual analysis. In J. Westwood, A. Gilroy, S. Linnell and T. McKenna (eds), *Art Therapy: Taking a Postcolonial, Aesthetic Turn*. The Netherlands: Sense, 230–251.

Thomson, J. 2019b. Wading in knee deep – the art therapist in different end-of-life settings. In M. Wood, R. Jacobson and H. Cridford (eds), *The Routledge Handbook of Art Therapy in Hospice and Bereavement Care*. London: Routledge, 185–198.

Thomson, J., Linnell, S., Laws, C. and Davies, B. 2018. Entanglements between art-making and storytelling in a collective biography on the death of an intimate other. *Departures in Critical Qualitative Inquiry*, 7(3), 4–26.

Wyatt, J. and Davies, B. 2011. Ethics. In Wyatt, J., Gale, K., Gannon, S. and Davies, B. (eds.), *Deleuze and Collaborative Writing: An Immanent Plane of Composition*. New York: Peter Lang, 105–129.

6

THREE COMPONENTS OF THE REFRAIN

> In which I explore the three interdependent components of the refrain: holding the world safe, establishing a safe plot of land, and, through a line of flight, throwing the world back into chaos. I explore the interdependence of these three components in everyday life, through the bird of paradise, through children's art and The Rite of Spring, and then through the simple act of leaving my apartment and going for a swim in an ocean pool one November morning.

In Chapter 5, I explored collective biography as a diffractive methodology, drawing on a story told at a collective biography workshop on the topic of death of an intimate other (Thomson et al., 2018). The story I chose carried a great deal of pain. In this chapter I turn from death to life lived to the full. I explore the ethico-onto-epistemology of refrains, where even inside repeated practice, the new is emergent: "The role of the imagination, or the mind which contemplates in its multiple and fragmented states, is to draw something new from repetition, to draw difference from it" (Deleuze, 2004: 97). Grøndahl (2000: 5) explores that moment of contemplation which draws something new from repetition. His protagonist wonders whether the "wearying commonplace everyday business" of life with small children has overshadowed the meaning of it all. But then he discovers, in the repetition, moments of ease that are as close as one gets to life's meaning:

> the meaning of it all was rather linked to the sum of repeated trivialities, the repetition itself, the patterns of repetition. While it was all going on I had only noticed it, the meaning, as a sudden and passing ease that could spread within me when, stumbling with exhaustion, I stopped midway between the

> kitchen table and the dishwasher with yet another dirty plate in my hand, hearing the children's laughter somewhere in the flat. Chance and isolated seconds, when it crossed my mind that precisely there, in transit through the repeated words and movements of the days and evenings, did I find myself in the midst of what had become my life, and that I should never get any closer to this centre.
>
> (Grøndahl, 2000: 5)

There is comfort too in repetition: "it conjures away the passage of time, the anxiety of death, the risk of chaos, the fear of losing control expressed by refrains, those rhythms that produce inhabited, territorialized time" (Dosse, 2010: 253). Those repetitions Deleuze and Guattari (1987) have theorised in terms of refrains; and refrains have three interdependent components or movements.

First, through their repetitions, or lines of descent, refrains hold the world safe; a repeated pattern wards off chaos (each morning we open the blinds, drink our coffee, get dressed, go out to face the day). We shape the territory we live within, in "rhythmic, melodious patterns, small chants, ditties, that shape the vibrations of milieus into the harmonics of territories, the organization of a wall or barrier" (Grosz, 2008: 54). The repetition of refrains offers "a kind of rhythmic regularity that brings a minimum of liveable order to a situation in which chaos beckons. It is the tapping of a kind of order of safety that protects the body through the rhythms of the earth itself" (Grosz, 2008: 52).

Never has our dependence on these small refrains, epistemological and ontological, been more visible to me, more tangible, than during the coronavirus lockdown. Daily routines such as walking around the Harbour, through the Botanic Garden and lying by the pond, are no longer possible. Sitting in the sun in my coffee shop reading over the last draft of a chapter is no longer possible. Kisses and hugs on greeting loved ones are no longer possible. Meeting friends and talking over dinner is no longer possible. My body struggles to re-inhabit itself in its solitude and uncertainty. I struggle to learn the new required habits of staying inside my flat, of endless handwashing, of creating distance between me and everyone else in my neighbourhood. My longing for my old routines, my old refrains, is visceral, aching. I depend on my "rhythmic, melodious patterns" much more than I realised…

Second, the refrain establishes a home, a safe plot of land. Walls and territories are created: it is "a circle of control that defines not only a safe inside but also a malleable or containable outside, a terrain to be marked, a field to be guarded (… a bird marks the field below its nest as the space of its sonorous and rhythmic performance)" (Grosz, 2008: 52). Humans are not alone in making territories that we mark and guard. Each morning, for example, the Australian bird of paradise

> cuts leaves, makes them fall to the ground, and turns them over so that the paler internal side contrasts with the earth. In this way it constructs a stage for itself like a ready-made; and directly above, on a creeper or branch, while

> fluffing its feathers beneath its beak to reveal their yellow roots, it sings a complex song made up from its own notes and, at intervals, those of other birds it imitates; it is a complete artist. This is not a synaesthesia of the flesh but blocs of sensations in the territory – colors, postures, and sounds that sketch out a total work of art. These sonorous blocs are refrains; but there are also refrains of posture and color, and postures and colors are always being introduced into refrains: bowing low, straightening up, dancing in a circle and a line of colours. The whole of the refrain is a being of sensation.
>
> (Deleuze and Guattari, 1994: 184)

Sound, movement, colour, each is integral to the bird's refrain, to the creation of its inner circle or territory, its zone of safety and the creation of a song that evolves in response to those other species who populate its outer territory. The children in Vuillard's painting, *Children in a room*, similarly create an inner circle or territory.

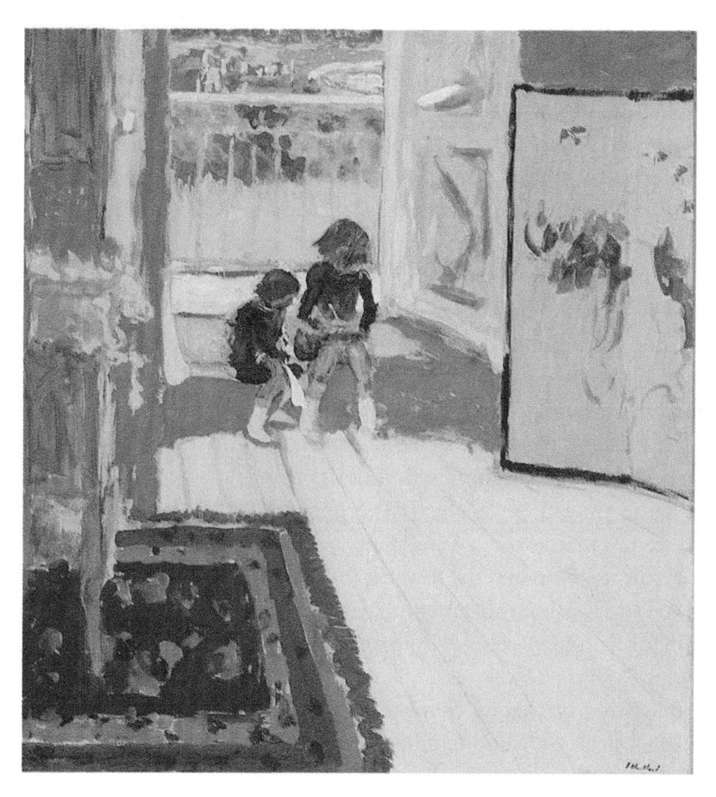

FIGURE 6.1 Jean-Edouard Vuillard, Children in a room (c. 1909).
Gouache on paper pasted on canvas. State Hermitage Museum, Saint Petersburg, Russia.

There is a small intimate circle around the girl who is drawing; her concentration is total as she makes her marks on the page. Her small sister, dressed in identical white boots and blue sailor suit, is captured in the safe circle of her concentration. She gazes at the movement of her sister's pencil. The "blocs of sensation in that territory ... sketch out a total work of art" (Deleuze and Guattari, 1994: 184). The girls sketch out a territory, as the bird of paradise does. The "total work of art" they sketch out is multi-layered; the work of art on the page, which is invisible to us, the circle of concentration that their artmaking creates around them, and the lines and colours, the blocs of sensation, that Vuillard has brought to his page, bringing the small circle of concentration to life for us, the viewers.

Vuillard's painting and our encounter with his painting form a palimpsest with children and their territory – one does not represent the other; one is not more real than the other; each is alive and lively. The girls, the painter, the viewer, the house, the paint materials are among the multiple entangled bodies that make up more-than-human life and liveliness. The girls create a territory, and in that territory is the possibility of change; Vuillard's painting, too, holds the possibility of change, which brings me to the third component of the refrain: "an experience of becoming, an experiential body of becoming, an experimentation producing new realities" (Zepke, 2005: 4).

This third component of the refrain is a de-territorialising break, or line of ascent through which the new emerges, which potentially throws the world back into chaos: "one opens the circle a crack, opens it all the way, lets someone in, calls someone, or else goes out oneself, launches forth" (Deleuze and Guattari, 1987: 311).

A line of flight opens up a glimpse of the not yet known: it is "a line of flight to the outside, a movement of migration, transformation, or deformation" (Grosz, 2008: 52). Far from being a representation of what already existed before Vuillard's painting, or before the encounter of the viewer with his painting, the *intra-action* among painter, viewer, children, and the materials used to make the painting, generates movements of "migration, transformation, or deformation" (Grosz, 2008: 52).

Finding life's meaning inside the repetition, creating new life through the making of territories, making art that both repeats and discovers, is transformative, a becoming, an experiment, a production of the new.

At the same time there is always the possibility of "'danger' inherent in any line that escapes, in any line of flight or creative deterritorialization: the danger of veering toward destruction, toward abolition" (Deleuze and Guattari, 1987: 299), a de-territorialising movement may be so small it is barely noticed, or it may afford a joyful, complex release from predictable, sometimes suffocating, repetitions (Davies, 2018).

The exploration of chaotic elements, the veering toward destruction, the abandonment of all that is safe and familiar is not always welcome. We come to depend on the sense of continuity – based on the belief that the current order can and will continue. That belief has been sorely tested in Australia, with the drought that went on for years, the rivers that dried up, the fires that burned, and then the coronavirus pandemic. The current talk, globally, about the climate emergency we are on the brink of, is anathema for those who hold grimly to the idea of the world as just, and orderly, and stable (Marshall, 2014). Their dependence on a sense of continuity may come with a deep antagonism to change, even in the arts.

Art in its various forms can protect us from chaos and release the new. Grosz is particularly interested in the transformative power of music:

> If the refrain protects us from chaos and entices us to abide and enjoy in a region provisionally enclosed from chaos, music opens up and transforms us, making of both our bodies and of the earth itself a new site of becomings toward a differently contained and directed chaos, to the opening up and exploration of chaotic elements.
>
> (Grosz, 2008: 56)

At the premiere of Stravinsky's *The Rite of Spring*, for example, the night began with the exquisite, much-loved ballet music by Chopin, *Les Sylphides*. The performance was "a reverie of romanticism, a work of pure poetic abstraction. Its only plot was its beauty" (Lehrer, 2007: 121). But then came the break. *The Rite* launched itself inside that same familiar romantic territory:

> After the applause faded, the auditorium filled with a pregnant pause ... At first *The Rite* is seductively easy. The tremulous bassoon, playing in its highest register (it sounds like a broken clarinet), echoes an old Lithuanian melody. To the innocent ear, this lilting tune sounds like a promise of warmth. Winter is over. We can hear the dead ground giving way to an arpeggio of green buds ... In one of music's most brutal transitions, Stravinsky opens the second section of his work with a monstrous migraine of sound ... Within seconds, the bassoon's flowery folk tunes are paved over by an epileptic rhythm, the horns colliding asymmetrically against the ostinato ... The tension builds and builds, but there is no vent ... This was when the audience at the premiere began to scream. *The Rite* had started a riot.
>
> (Lehrer, 2007: 122)

Eventually, as it was repeated, *The Rite* lost its power to disturb; the listeners got used to it. As Lehrer says, "Nothing is difficult forever" (Lehrer, 2007: 125). The line of descent absorbs the line of ascent, modifying itself as it does so. If all we have are the simple repetitions, we risk growing bored, and crave the presence of the third movement of the refrain – the line of flight – the break.

What I pursue in what follows, through a slice of my life one Spring morning, is the *complex interdependence* of the three components.

Life does not move from one component of the refrain to another; it is never simply this or that component, never either/or. As Grosz observes, "Every refrain is marked by all three aspects or movements" (2008: 52–53).

The swim

I begin this story in the charmed circle of my fourth-story inner-city flat. That inner circle is replete with the satisfying thing-power of my books and artworks – and all the precious things I have collected and lived with for decades. While the concept of charmed circle usually refers to a group of people who have special power or influence, and do not allow anyone else to join their group, I am using it here to refer first to my flat and its things, and then the six-storey Art Deco building that contains my flat. The flat and the building are active agents, which have power and influence in the task of containing the people who reside here, protecting them from chaos.

I begin my morning with yoga and pilates on my living room floor. I am bathed in early morning light; alone, the sun and I, and blue sky, its clouds backlit with morning sun, blinding gold on their puffed edges, deep blue grey in their centres. I shut my eyes for a few moments against the blinding light. I am listening to Gluck's *Orphée et Eurydice*. Glorious voices intertwined with the backlit clouds. Orpheus's longing for Eurydice is intense, and unbearable. Outside my window the rainbow lorikeets swoop and chortle, provoked by the music.

A quick breakfast, lovingly prepared before I settled into my exercise routine, and it's time to venture out of my nest:

> One launches forth, hazards an improvisation. But to improvise is to join with the World, or meld with it. One ventures from home on the thread of a tune. Along sonorous, gestural, motor lines that mark the customary path … and graft themselves onto or begin to bud 'lines of drift' with different loops, knots, speeds, movements, gestures, and sonorities.
>
> (Deleuze and Guattari, 1987: 311–312)

Back-pack on, I unlock the heavy wooden door and push it open into the second layer of my charmed circle. Tap, tap, tap down four flights of stairs. On the ground floor is Mabel, just turned three, sitting near the front door with her scooter. "Hello Mabel," I say, "you have your beautiful new scooter with you." She smiles up at me. "And you have something else," I say, looking at a jewel-encrusted box tucked behind her scooter. "What?" she asks, surprised. I point to the box. "Oh," she says and picks it up and holds it out to show me. "What have you got in it," I ask. She takes off the lid and shows me her treasures, explaining what each one is. She puts the lid on carefully and asks me where I'm going. "To swim", I tell her. "To Bondi, to Icebergs swimming pool." Her mother joins us and tells Mabel they can go to Bondi when her swimming improves. "The baby pool is especially lovely at Icebergs," I tell her, "she would love it." "We must go she says," a little doubtful, then, "we *must* go," she says, more definite this time, and adds," I'm reading your book. I've enrolled in an M.Teach, and I've made your book my preliminary reading."

I am surprised and touched. This second layer of my charmed circle is very precious to me.

I step outside into Springfield Ave, down the steps and along the path into the back lane that goes down to the station. It has started raining lightly. Someone is cocooned in blankets, asleep in an alcove in the back wall of one of the buildings. This neighbourhood, is, curiously, a third charmed circle, though the multiple layers of territories cross over each other in a more visible way. The locals are protective of the homeless and the aged. When Sydney's Mayor promised to 'cleanse' the area of street people, the locals were outraged and told her in passionate public speeches to back off. Further down the lane an ice (methamphetamine/crystal meth) addict is rummaging through garbage bins searching for treasures; he has spread his finds over the pavement and on to the street in a crazed mimicry of the bird of paradise. But there is no sonorous and rhythmic performance to follow, as far as I can tell. With the matter that the owners of the bins have abjected, the ice addict creates his territory, making himself safe with a pattern that is familiar, but perhaps also opening up for himself something new in his work of art, "a movement of migration, transformation, or deformation" (Grosz, 2008: 52), something that may be both exciting and dangerous, "veering toward destruction, toward abolition" (Deleuze and Guattari, 1987: 299). And later, perhaps days later, the city council's street cleaners will clear away the abandoned mess.

I dodge some dog poo. Someone who depends on their small dog to make their charmed circle safe has forgotten to bring their plastic poo bag. Or maybe it was just too hard for old joints to bend down and pick it up. Or maybe it was an act of territorialisation. Maybe this is the area the dog owner claims as theirs for their dog's doings, and perhaps they choose not to litter the world with yet more plastic bags...

I turn the corner, down two flights of stairs, glance up at the screen, train to Bondi Junction due in two minutes. Running now, slap my Opal card on to the sensor, *kping!*, gate flies open, run through and down the escalator, immobile passengers to the left, those in a hurry to the right. The train thunders, moans and hisses into the station, and the doors open with a high-pitched moan. The passengers spill out, and the stream of new passengers boards the train. A series of rapid, high-pitched hoots and the doors close. Each passenger settles down into a small charmed circle, half of them immersed in intimate engagement with their phones, the others staring into inner space. I gaze out of the windows, hoping to see the jacarandas newly in bloom, spreading their violet light through the city, as they do each November.

After the stop at Edgecliff I turn to my newspaper. Dirt has been unearthed on our "accidental" prime minister, Scott Morrison, the man whom nobody knows, and who claims to have played no part in engineering the coup. Apparently, his church secured him the position by fasting and praying – though he knew nothing of it, being loyal to the old PM to the last, and having, he declared, no plan to displace him. Now it seems he was fired from his last job for dodgy dealings. I read: "Scott Morrison could be described as Trump Lite plus a combination of toe-curling folksiness, condescension and religiosity. Like Trump he is fundamentally incurious. On issues raised with him, he either knows the answers already, or has no desire to hear the case for and against a proposition" (Jones, 2018: 7). He is also, like Trump, blithely willing to contradict himself as if that poses no problem and requires no justification. They're not lies, apparently; he is just carrying out his job. The train roars into Bondi Junction, hissing and hooting.

A long queue forms at the 333 bus stop; orderly, mostly quiet, except for some tourists who shout to each other, establishing their own territory in an unfamiliar landscape. The bus arrives and a hundred or more people climb on, the only sound over the engine's burr, the rhythmic *kping!* of the Opal cards tapping on.

I turn again to my paper. The situation of the refugee children on Nauru is dire. The doctors, desperate to get medical help for them, are constantly denied. Some doctors have lost their jobs for telling the Australian public the truth of what is going on, on the island. Now a small child has life-threatening sepsis, and probably meningitis, but the Australian border force doesn't give a damn. It refuses permission for the child to get treatment. It takes court order after court order to counteract its wilful indifference.

How has my country become so brutal, so profoundly unethical? What refrains do the politicians use to convince themselves and the 'general public' that their inhumanity is normal, even desirable? The new evangelical prime minister, Scott Morrison, was the minister instrumental in designing the harsh Australian border protection policies. He proudly displays in his office a block of metal in the shape of an abstract Asian fishing boat sailing on an abstract wave, on which is painted in thick black letters, the boast "I stopped these". When asked how this trophy accords with his evangelical Christianity, he says his Christian values are his business, and he had simply been doing his job.

The bus pulls over at the Bondi Beach stop, doors swing open, rhythmic kping! of people tapping off. Down the footpath, press the traffic-light button, wait, click, click, click; a stream of humans crosses the road and surges down to beach or pool. At the pool I hold out my pool card, wait for a hole to be snipped in it, and I'm through the gate. I change in the women's changing room, leave my things neatly folded, then down the steps and into the ice-cold, pale-blue pool with its white-painted surfaces and black-painted lines and ropes that mark off the lanes. I slide into the cold velvet of ice-blue water.

I make for my favourite lane where the ocean waves crash over the edge when the tide and the swell are high enough, in a roaring, rhythmic disruption of the calm surface of the pool: an interface between order and chaos. The pool, perched on the edge of the ocean, is a circle of control; it defines a safe inside, right next to the uncontrollable outside – the great, green, rolling, thundering, spuming Pacific Ocean.

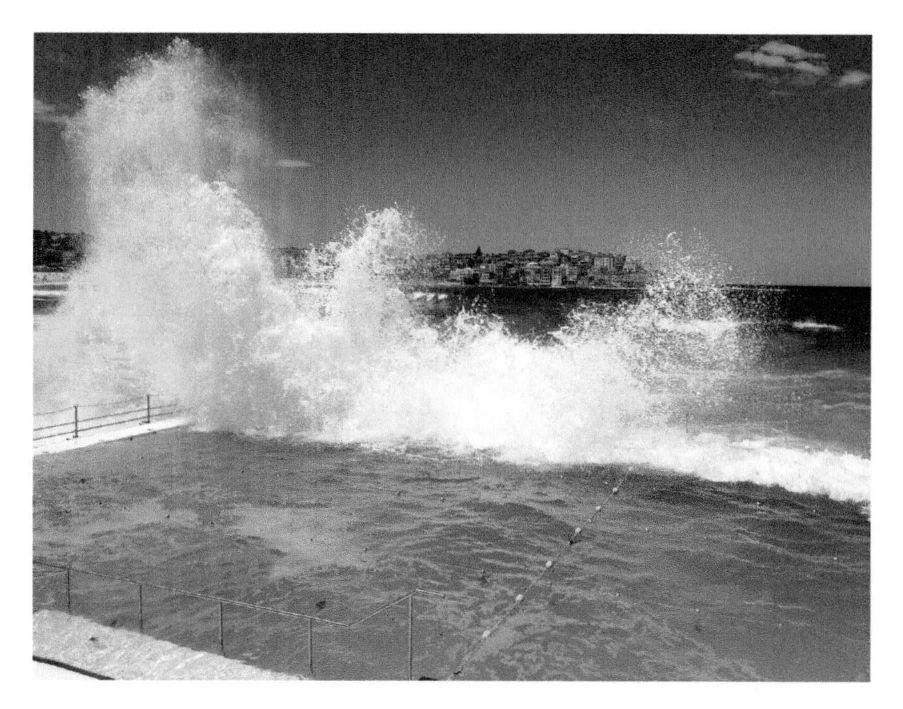

FIGURE 6.2 Icebergs swimming pool at high tide.
Bondi, NSW. Photograph by Bronwyn Davies, 2018.

Inside each lane, the swimmers swim on the left in an orderly chain, each swimming along the appropriate black line. And I'm in luck. There is a man in my lane who swims beautifully. And another, a "thrasher" I think rather uncharitably. As I settle into my swim, my strokes absorb the smooth rhythm and strength of the beautiful swimmer. I am transported, outside the realm of everyday life even inside the repetitive movement of swimming. The in-breath under my left, raised arm, reveals a bright flash of blue sky streaked with glorious clouds like fish scales, the waves rhythmically roar and crash against the outside of the pool, the expelled air from my lungs has a different beat as it bubbles past my ears. My hands slide soundlessly under the water, creating a rhythmic stream of light-filled bubbles. Every few minutes a series of three waves smashes against the pool wall, spattering sharp drops of foam on to my back and sending waves rollicking across the surface of the pool. The rocking of the waves and the spattering of the foam ties me to the moon and the wind and the time of day – the earth element of my swimming refrain.

Two twittering, plump-breasted bikini-clad girls take over a corner of the pool, squealing at their own daring whenever the waves splash them. With their waterproof camera, they take shots of each other for Facebook, or whichever platform it is that has territorialised them, providing what they hope is their safe space.

Suddenly, inexplicably, at the end of a lap, the beautiful swimmer has stopped in front of me. I pull up startled. He says sorry. It's ok, I say, and add, you're a beautiful swimmer. Thank you, he says, and I take off on my next lap, worrying that I have opened a small space he might misinterpret. Then another refrain overlaps it and overtakes it: what will happen if someone makes off with my back-pack? How will I get home on the bus and the train in my wet swimmers and bare feet and no Opal card? I am dogged for a minute with an all too familiar, unbearable sense of vulnerability, felt vividly in my body; a vulnerability that arises, for any of us, when we become aware of the hairsbreadth distance between safety and chaos. I go back to the safety of the rhythms, sinking back into breath and movement and the pale-blue water washing over me.

The bikini-clad girls are in the pool now, swimming the wrong way up the lane. Luckily, it's too cold for them. They just need a couple of underwater shots, boobs afloat.

They leave, and I relax back into the slow, rhythmic movement, in sync once more with the beautiful swimmer, the waves, the ocean, the sky and the clouds. Inside that repetition, lap after lap, I become fish, water sliding over silver scales, languid body gliding, mouth now a gill, and the fish-scaled sky above. "These rhythms of the body ... coupled with those of the earth – seasons, tides, temperatures – are the conditions of the refrain, which encapsulates and abstracts these rhythmic or vibratory forces into a sonorous emblem, a composed rhythm" (Grosz, 2008: 55).

At the end of 45 minutes, according to the pool clock, I linger in the water, gazing out over beach, rocks and headland, and the green, foam-capped waves.

In the changing room my bag sits orderly and undisturbed, waiting for me. I revel in the hot shower, thawing out cold limbs, becoming-human once more as I rub warm-bloodedness back into them. The glorious roar of the waves is magnified in the cubicle of the shower, resonating through my body; I am vibrating with the force of the cosmos.

On the train on the way home, each human, as usual, is encapsulated in their own bubble. Then a voice at the front of the carriage loudly addresses us, drawing us together in surprise, as one listening organism.

> *Hello everyone. I am sorry to bother you but I didn't know where else to go. My name is Rory. I know it's really annoying when people ask you for money. I'm just trying to scrape a few dollars together. My mum and dad can't help me. They've got nothing. My brother's got nothing. I'm really sorry to bother you. I've got nowhere to go. I wonder if you could help me.*

The carriage is frozen to attention, held in his plea – and in our seats. We can't walk on as we might have done in the street, where most likely we would not have heard the words he had rehearsed. As the train carries us safely to home or to work, Rory has nowhere to go. This is a radical departure from the usual refrains of begging; "one opens the circle a crack, opens it all the way, lets someone in, calls someone, or else goes out oneself, launches forth" (Deleuze and Guattari, 1987: 311). Rory has a name and a family who has abandoned him. And nowhere to go. In my head is the usual, familiar refrain: you should not give to beggars, they will only spend your money on drugs or alcohol. Each time I refuse one of them, chanting that familiar refrain to myself, my heart freezes over. Each time it does, I reassure myself with another refrain: that social security and the charities I regularly give money to, will work out how best to help them. But I always feel sick in my refusal. Now, no one moves, no one can move, and Rory continues to stand there, looking at us, waiting. The carriage has become his territory, the passengers are compelled by his plea and held together as one in his gaze. I have $5 in my backpack – that is all I ever take with me to the pool. Overriding the refrain that says wrong, stupid, gullible, I unzip my pack and hold the pink five-dollar note out to him. He takes it and thanks me, but I can't look in his eyes for the shame I feel at his having to beg from me. Hands along the length of the carriage hold out money and he politely thanks each one and moves on. Relief sweeps through the carriage; a small crack has opened – a gesture rippling against the tide of inhumanity that constantly washes over us.

The money could solve very little in Rory's life; and we had each been given the chance to engage in kindness toward a stranger, recovering for that brief moment, our own humanity. I sit lost in contemplation of Rory's story and of the collective response. The train hisses and roars into Kings Cross station, and we stream out of the door forming the familiar two lines, one standing still on the left-hand side, being lifted up, and the other, of which I am part, taking pleasure in walking up the escalator. And I am home, walking up Springfield Ave to my apartment building, and when I unlock the door and walk in, loving the beauty and calm of its wood-panelled lobby and hallway. I walk up the four flights of stairs and I am home. I hang up my towel and swimmers to dry in the bathroom and head out to the café with my notebook and pencil. I sit in the sun, order my morning piccolo, and begin writing this chapter.

A week later, returning from my swim, this time seated at the front of the carriage, Rory appeared again, arresting everyone's attention. I was close behind him this time, not caught in his gaze. He hadn't spent his windfall on a bath. His spiel was identical to last time. The words that had offered us our own humanity now sounded false. Why ply the same trail, I wondered, and risk meeting the same people who will come to hear your words as a scam? But his words had the same effect as last time – hands held out, offering him money. He has hit on a refrain that works well. I was affronted at discovering yet again my own gullibility, but also impressed. I was not held in his gaze this time, and thus not part of the territory he commanded with his gaze and his plea. I no longer felt compelled to repeat my earlier small act of kindness and the refrain that categorised him as a scammer took over. The woman across the aisle from me, also behind Rory and out of his gaze, shrugged helplessly and we smiled at each other, wryly, void of answers.

Rory's refrain may have been the only words he knew to keep him safe, and they were also a radical departure on more usual begging refrains. It seems such an obvious mistake to repeat the routine so precisely, on the same train at the same time. Was his daring so great that he could only bring himself to travel the same train line that produced money last time? If his refrain brought him the "rhythmic regularity that brings a minimum of liveable order to a situation in which chaos beckons" (Grosz, 2008: 52) then it makes sense that he tried to repeat it precisely as he had done it before. Is his refrain, for that matter, any different from Prime Minister Morrison's – a man 'just doing his job', figuring how to survive against the odds, given the rapid turnover of Australian prime ministers? Or mine, as I territorialise the pool in a repeated refrain that gives me a liveable order on the edge of chaos?

References

Davies, B. 2018. Encounters with difference and the entangled enlivening of being. *Departures in Critical Qualitative Research*, 7(4), 1–19.

Deleuze, G. 2004. *Difference and Repetition* (trans. P. Patton). London: Continuum.

Deleuze, G. and Guattari, F. 1994. *What Is Philosophy?* (trans. H. Tomlinson and G. Burchell). New York: Columbia University Press.

Deleuze, G. and Guattari, F. 1987. *A Thousand Plateaus: Capitalism and Schizophrenia* (trans. B. Massumi). Minneapolis, MN: University of Minnesota Press.

Dosse, F. 2010. *Gilles Deleuze and Felix Guattari: Intersecting Lives* (trans. D. Glassman). Chichester, UK: Columbia University Press.

Grosz, E. 2008. *Chaos, Territory, Art, Deleuze and the Framing of the Earth*. New York: Columbia University Press.

Grøndahl, J. C. 2000. *Silence in October* (trans. A. Born). Melbourne, Vic: Text Publishing.

Jones, B. 2018. Saving planet earth. *The Saturday Paper*, 10–16 November, no. 230, 9.

Lehrer, J. 2007. *Proust Was a Neuroscientist*. New York: Houghton Mifflin Company.

Marshall, G. 2014. *Don't Even Think About It*. London: Bloomsbury.

Thomson, J., Linnell, S., Laws, C. and Davies, B. 2018. Entanglements between art-making and storytelling in a collective biography on the death of an intimate other. *Departures in Critical Qualitative Inquiry*, 7(3), 4–26.

Vuillard, J.-E. 1934. *Children in a room*. Moscow: State Museum of New Western Art.

Zepke, S. 2005. *The Abstract Machine: Art and Ontology in Deleuze and Guattari*. New York: Routledge.

7
RECOGNITION

> In which I explore the concept and practice of recognition, analysing it in terms of three interdependent components: affirming normativity through possession; forming borders through dispossessing the other; and creative–relational affirmation of difference. I explore the act of recognition in encounters within human and more-than-human lives.

In Chapter 6, I turned from death to life lived to the full, through the ethico-onto-epistemology of refrains. Even inside repeated practice, the new emerges. I told the story of Rory, and the way a carriage full of people responded to his plea for recognition. I want to explore further here the complex links between humanity – in the sense of the best that humans, and more-than-humans are capable of – and recognition.

Recognition is a concept not much loved by new materialist philosophers because of its strong connection with identity politics, which individualise on the one hand, and on the other limit each subject to their identity category. It is argued that while the point in "turning to recognition is often to value difference, the risk is of complicity with regimes of visibility. In this way, recognition becomes coded as that which is visible and articulable and what is beyond recognition is rendered invisible" (Stark, 2017: 103). Deleuze claimed at least once that "recognition has never sanctioned anything but the recognizable and the recognized; form will never inspire anything but conformities" (Deleuze, 1994: 134). Grosz went further in her opposition to the concept of recognition, suggesting that "the whole ethical predication based upon recognition of the other should be purely and simply abandoned" (Grosz, 2001: 25). She claimed that recognition "is the force of conservatism, the tying of the new and the never-conceived to that which is already cognized"

(Grosz, 2001: 103). New materialist thought-action seeks to focus on the emergence of difference, on differenciation, and on the thinking and doing that facilitates our becoming other than we were. It values lines of flight and the emergence of the not-yet-thought:

> The power of the line of flight is that it provides an escape route from established patterns and coherences. The line of flight is creative and experimental; it is not concerned with coding or overcoding but with mutation. This is not about the great ruptures in systems but "the little crack, the imperceptible ruptures" which enable lines of flight to slip into gaps, everywhere.
>
> (Stark, 2017: 91, citing Deleuze and Parnet, 2007: 131)

I *re-turn* to recognition, here, not abandoning it, or trapped in its forms, but to think about it, further, as movement. To do this I work with Massumi's concept of sympathy and Barad's concept of response-ability: "Responding – being responsible/response-able – to the thick tangles of spacetimematterings that are threaded through us, the places and times from which we came but never arrived and never leave, is perhaps what *re-turning* is about" (Barad, 2014: 184).

My interest in the concept-practice of recognition has been provoked for some time by the surprising rush of tears to my eyes when I witness a heartfelt acknowledgement of one person by another, particularly when what is being recognised is extraordinary, or what Massumi (2015) would call supernormal. That celebratory act of recognition overrides the inertia of normality and its accompanying resistance to change. The affective flow in that act both surprises and affects me. I find myself moved in and by encounters between strangers, caught up in the flow in-between. Becoming part of that flow in-between releases me momentarily from ordinariness, from the press toward the repetition of the same, and from the isolation that characterises so much of the human(ist) condition.

My other provocation to re-turn to recognition is the global increase in the refusal of recognition, when someone (or some group) is refused recognition and made unrecognisable as human, unworthy of those usual forms of recognition granted to others. There is a lot of that refusal going on in Australia at the moment, with politicians refusing to recognise the original custodians of this land, or to recognise refugees, or the poor, who are treated with contempt and forced to live in barely survivable conditions (Davies, 2018, 2019). And while the position of women is structurally better than it was in the 1970s and 1980s, contempt for and abuse of women is everywhere, as it is for the disabled. With the advent of the coronavirus pandemic in 2020 all these failures of recognition are becoming painfully more evident, with the "aged" getting repeated special mention – their category membership re-cognised as warranting different treatment, making it more likely they will be locked in, deprived of social support, or left to die.

I explore, in this chapter, *three interconnected components of recognition. The first, recognition as possession,* arises from, and confirms, the normative social order. It possesses and is possessed by the normative order, and it happens fast like a spring recoiling. *The second component* is *recognition as dispossession/dis-recognition.* This also affirms the normative order through the simultaneous acts of self-possession and dispossession of another. The dispossessed other is used to create the safe borders of the normative social order. *The third component, recognition as creative-relationality*, celebrates a break from normative assemblages through encounters in which the unexpected and the new becomes recognisable and worthy of being valued. Deleuze observes of creative-relational encounters that we have not sufficiently valued them, having "preferred the facility of recognitions" (Deleuze, 2000: 27) by which he means, I think, recognition as possession.

In new materialist thought, we are each more-than-human subjects-in-relation who emerge, not as separate or complete entities *in* the world, but as entangled becomings *of* the world: "To be entangled is not simply to be intertwined with another, as in the joining of separate entities, but to lack an independent, self-contained existence" (Barad, 2007: ix). Recognising the specificity, the singularity, of another's emergence in that entangled becoming, is not a simple matter of acknowledging someone who is already formed. Recognition enables the possibility of one another's existence in the world's emergent becoming: "We become-with each other or not at all," wrote Haraway (2016: 4). Individual and world are co-constitutive and co-emergent. Recognition is not an optional extra.

The approach to becoming that I explore here offers a marked departure from Butler's dual dynamic of subordination to often unwanted and unacknowledged terms, and the dependence on those same terms:

> Let us consider that a subject is not only formed in subordination, but that this subordination provides the subject's continuing condition of possibility... The child does not know to what he/she attaches; yet the infant as well as the child must attach in order to persist in and as itself. No subject can emerge without this attachment, formed in dependency, but no subject, in the course of its formation, can ever fully afford to "see" it.
>
> (Butler, 1997: 8)

In this chapter I look at what we find hard (or cannot fully afford) to "see".

I explore the ways in which acts of recognition, and the *terms of recognition themselves*, are necessarily emergent. The term and the practices of recognition are integral to the multiple and often contradictory processes of becoming-with- and becoming-of-the-world. They are at the same time enabling and disabling, but always needing to be worked on and worked over.

That working over sometimes becomes highly visible, demanding major ethico-onto-epistemological reconfigurations, such as in the AIDs crisis or the current coronavirus pandemic. Such reconfigurations of our habituated entanglements can be confronting and confusing. Yet habituated, repeated acts of recognition run the risk of losing their vitality.

A problem with habituation, Doerr (2007: 54) wrote, is that we lose sensation and with it our capacity to see:

> To eat a banana for the thousandth time is nothing like eating a banana for the first time. To have sex with somebody for the thousandth time is nothing like having sex with that person for the first time. The easier an experience, or the more entrenched, or the more familiar, the fainter our sensation of it becomes. This is true of chocolate and marriages and hometowns and narrative structures. Complexities wane, miracles become unremarkable, and if we're not careful, pretty soon we're gazing out at our lives as if through a burlap sack.

Yet even in habituated repetitions, as I explored in Chapter 6, the new emerges: "The role of the imagination, or the mind which contemplates in its multiple and fragmented states, is to draw something new from repetition, to draw difference from it" (Deleuze, 2004: 97).

Recognition, then, is not a matter of a pre-existing entity affirming, or failing to affirm, another pre-existing entity. And the terms of recognition are not simply an oppressive, unchanging weight that dictates what we are and can be – though it is sometimes that. They are also emergent and evolving, always changing. Further, acts of recognition cannot *fix* the object of the gaze, though they are often spoken about as if they do just that. An unwavering gaze, as Doerr points out, diminishes its object; the more we recognise someone or something as the same, the more we lose sight/taste/sound/feel of them, of their multiplicity, and their emergence in relation to others both human and more-than-human.

In a Cartesian or Enlightenment imagination, the individual is permanently isolated, unable to know the other, or be known, since the gap between self and other is unbridgeable. Individuals caught up in that perspective expend a great deal of energy reflexively examining themselves – or, more accurately, trying to find a self to examine. The empathy that therapists are exhorted to engage in, involves an attempt to stand in the shoes of the other as they struggle to find that examinable self (Wyatt, 2019). From a new materialist perspective, in contrast, the act of recognition involves an entanglement of multiple, emergent subjects, an entanglement that is constitutive of the ethical matter and mattering of the world's enfolding and unfolding. Rather than an unbridgeable gap between self and other, extracting oneself from the multiple, more-than-human lines of force, is, in new materialist thought, virtually impossible.

The third component, recognition as creative-relationality, occurs when we are open to what is different and new. It depends on *sympathy*, a creative emotion like love or joy. While intuition is an intimate relation of a being with itself, sympathy reaches *through* intuition towards a reality outside itself; "it reaches the material in matter, the vital in living forms, the social in societies, the personal in individual existences" (Lapoujade, 2019: np). Through sympathy we become more-than-ourselves – we exceed ourselves – we go beyond habituated knowing in being, and engage in what Bergson calls creative evolution, and Nancy (2007, 2017) calls world-becoming.

The trouble for those whose desire is to hold everything the same through acts of recognition such as possession and dispossession, is that knowing in being is necessarily multiple, emergent and evolving, and the terms of recognition inevitably change. *Identities* may be threatened by those changes, since each identity depends on the terms of recognition through which it gained its "identity". This is the ethico-onto-epistemological dilemma that lies at the heart of recognition.

As I write, there are people around the world marching in the Black Lives Matter protest in defiance of orders not to congregate and in defiance of the deadly virus. Identities constructed around beliefs in white supremacy are threatened by such mass calls for change and they attempt to lock in, not just people in their homes, but the categories and beliefs that maintain their dominance. Even those who recognise that change is desirable can fight back against the tide of change (Davies and Harré, 1990).

The struggle that changing terms of recognition involve was evident at the inquest into the death in custody of Tanya Day, an Australian indigenous woman. Her family's barrister, Peter Morrissey SC, grilled the witness, Superintendent Sussan Thomas, on her understanding of "unconscious bias":

> "Well..." Thomas, her dark hair pulled into a tight ponytail, starts slowly. "My understanding is that we all have, um, from our experiences and from our cultural upbringings ... opinions or views, unconscious to ourselves, not at the forefront of our minds, and it can impact on the way we think."
>
> In a landmark ruling, Coroner Caitlin English has agreed to consider whether systemic racism, and therefore "opinions or views unconscious", were a contributing factor in Day's death.
>
> (Hooper, 2019–20: 61)

Superintendent Thomas was the most senior officer to give evidence on the final day of the court hearings. She was someone who had gone out of her way to confront racism in herself and in the force. She had been responsible for the development of a training package on indigenous cultural awareness for Victorian Police, had been to an Indigenous cultural awareness camp, and oversaw the publication of Aboriginal fact sheets that were available to any officer who sought them. Hooper continues her account of the hearing:

> "You're aware that the Royal Commission into Aboriginal Deaths in Custody released its findings 30 years ago?" Morrissey asks Thomas.
>
> "Yes." She graduated from the Victoria Police Academy in 1989.
>
> "You accept that Aboriginal people continue to have disproportionate contact with the justice system?"
>
> "Yes."
>
> "You accept that Aboriginal women are 24 times more likely to be imprisoned than non-Aboriginal women?"

> "I do know there's an over-representation."
>
> "Do you accept that Aboriginal people continue to disproportionately die in custody?"
>
> "Yes, I'm familiar with statistics that suggest that."
>
> The superintendent, her collar buttoned to the top, is holding herself erect, but her face is red with tension. One imagines her frustration at being served up as the inquest's sacrificial offering co-mingling with the defensiveness police feel about being called on to justify themselves to lawyers who don't work on the ugly frontline, and whose own motives and biases are never questioned. Perhaps she can reasonably feel aggrieved that, as an agent of change and good deeds, she's being treated suddenly as an ignoramus and a bigot.
>
> (Hooper, 2019–20: 63)

Superintendent Thomas worked in a system whose biases are so habituated that all of her work toward change has apparently had little effect on the practices that lead to the deaths in custody of the original custodians of the land. Tanya Day was arrested for drunkenness. She was causing no offence to anyone, yet her condition was reported by another passenger on the train to the engine driver who reported it to the police who were waiting at the station to arrest her and place her in a cell. Non-indigenous people who are drunk in public are more likely to be ignored, or if they are intercepted, driven home. Indeed, one of my sons was driven home when he fell down dead drunk in public, late at night. The policeman who drove him home sympathised with my horror at the sight of my bedraggled, vomity teenaged son, who I had thought was safely tucked up in bed. In extraordinary contrast, the lines of descent when it comes to racial bias are hard to shift. Even Thomas, at the forefront of change, could not bring herself to *see* that:

> "You don't dispute that adult humans are affected by unconscious bias, do you?"
>
> "No, I don't," acknowledges Thomas.
>
> "Do you accept that systemic racism does persist in the justice system?"
>
> "No." She is quietly spoken now, dry-throated. "I'm not in a position to answer that question."
>
> "Why is that?"
>
> "Because in my 30 years of policing, I haven't had that experience."
>
> The audience gasps. As public theatre, the less woke the witness's answers the better.
>
> "Do you accept that systemic racism and discrimination persists within Victoria Police?"
>
> Thomas is flushed but utterly still. "No. No, I don't."
>
> The laughter from the Indigenous people present is bitter: what exactly did she learn on cultural awareness camp?
>
> (Hooper, 2019–20: 63)

The Victoria Police cannot be *seen* by Superintendent Thomas to be racist in this context, despite the overwhelming evidence of incarceration and deaths in custody to the contrary. *Not seeing*, despite apparently recognising the need for change, is in part to do with maintaining the terms of recognition, and in part with a failure of sympathy for the systemically dispossessed.

Without sympathy each of us is capable of abhorrent acts of dispossession. Such acts of dispossession are, of course, not limited to the police force. In 2013, Australian football crowds were swept up in loud, relentless booing, intended to destroy the footballer Adam Goodes. The sound they made every time Goodes took possession of the ball was like a jet plane taking off. They kept it up all season and continued into the next. Goodes was an indigenous football player, regarded as the greatest AFL (Australian rules football) player in a generation. In 2014 he became Australian of the Year, a position he was awarded for his work on reconciliation and his calls for an end to racism.

In the beginning he had been the football fans' beloved possession, winning the highest order of medals for his exceptional play. His indigeneity was forgiven and forgotten. He excelled in a way no other players had ever done, and they loved him for it. As fans they collectively joined in his brilliance on the field – they participated in it, enlarging themselves and enlarging him in their mutual responsiveness. But when he objected to racist name-calling from one of the fans, they turned against him. Every effort was, in repeated acts of brutal mass hysteria, turned toward his dispossession (Grant, 2019).

In German there is a word we don't have in English: *Zersetzung,* meaning breakdown, decomposition, degradation (Funder, 2019–20). The fans were intent on Goodes' *Zersetzung*; people who knew him reported that his heart was broken by the repeated chanting aimed at bringing that about.

Belief and the terms of recognition

Recognisable specificity, or identity, has, in everyday common sense (that is, the Enlightenment or Cartesian sense), been interpreted as being emergent from *within* the individual, albeit with some help from parents, guardians and teachers – and sometimes, too, the animals we've formed relations with. That common sense is misleading; what we are does not arise from within with a little help from outside. We are formed in our always emergent specificity and multiplicity in relation to others, human others and more-than-human others. Those others include the land we live on, the food and shelter the land provides, as well as its changing climatic conditions (Davies, 2018). The common-sense view makes it difficult to see the force of the more-than-human entanglements through which we are made, and make ourselves, recognisable. And so we mistake the source of our knowing in being, and we marshal moral frameworks that elevate and reinforce the ascendance of our individualistic, humanist selves, and their familiar terms of recognition.

Individuals' (collective) beliefs, through which they are identified, do not, as we tend to assume, *belong* to them alone. Belief, rather, signals life-qualities held in relation to others, that holding-in-relation being fundamental to sympathy – and sympathy is fundamental to the holding-in-common of the human animal:

> belief is a 'possession'. It is the possession of a multiplicity of life-qualities by *each other* ... In Bergsonian terms, this immediate possession of life qualities by each other can be considered a primary sympathy … [Sympathy] is a self-effecting qualitative movement constitutive of the life of the animal. *The animal does not have sympathy; it is sympathy.*
>
> (Massumi, 2015: 10–11)

And to the extent that this is so, the withdrawal of sympathy, or the ambivalent, ambiguous contraction of sympathy, can be life-threatening, as it was for Tanya Day, for Goodes, for refugees, for the poor, the aged, the disabled, and for indigenous people, both children and adults. That lack of sympathy was extended to me, and by me in return, in the early days of the 2020 coronavirus shutdown. I remonstrated with a middle-aged man who refused to allow me any space to pass him on a narrow pathway. I first pinned myself against the rock wall on the side of the path, imagining it as a signal for him to move over to the other side of the path. As he stared at me and walked deliberately toward me I scrambled backwards up on to a small ledge in the sheer vertical wall behind me, and expostulated at his selfishness. "Go fuck yourself, you old hag" he shouted as he swaggered on aggressively up the middle of the path.

What the pandemic does is throw usual forms of recognition into disarray, disrupting even the everyday forms of courtesy among strangers. Unlike the strangers on the train intra-acting with Rory in Chapter 6, neither I nor the swaggering middle-aged man had any humanity left in that encounter. What we once, perhaps, possessed in common no longer held.

Let me return to my three components of recognition in light of this discussion so far.

Recognition as possession

The first component of recognition takes place in acts of sympathetic possession-in-common. It is generated and maintained through the reiteration of collective beliefs and actions, through which subjects are possessed. We develop "a sense of ourselves of, in and as assemblages" (Harris et al., 2019: np). That predictable, reiterable sense of ourselves gives us, and others, recognisable "identities". Through that possession individuals become (more or less) predictable and recognisable as themselves in relation to each other.

This first component takes place within a predictable, repetitive assemblage of shared knowing in being. A *recognisable* self and other are made possible by reiteration within that assemblage. Reiteration generates a functional world – including human subjects with their identifiable sense of self – as if the world were objectifiably knowable, rather than relationally emergent: "Recognition takes recursive return for identity. It constrains recurrence to the same" (Massumi, 2015: 13). That constraining can work with or against creative-relationality, the third component of recognition. The reiterated world creates a sense of safety and stability, and it creates what we think of, and recognise, as normality, which allows the world to function.

Recognition as dispossession/dis-recognition: An exclusion that matters

The reiterated assemblage that possesses, and makes a safe space for those who possess and are possessed, denies that safe space to others, dispossessing them, denying them recognition as human within its terms. Dispossession takes place when sympathetic relationality is shut down, effectively denying the safety of familiar positionings previously or otherwise held by those dispossessed. It creates borders inside which the possessed can go on recognising themselves and others, taking their own identities to be stable and their terms of recognition to be superior; they abject the other who is different (Shildrick, 2002). Australia's Border Force, the systemic assemblage that keeps asylum seekers, who come by boat, out of Australia, is aptly named.

These two components of recognition, possession and dispossession, do not operate as a binary. They work in tandem; one might submit to the terms of the normative order, making its terms one's own, only to find oneself marginalised and excoriated within those same terms, as was the footballer Adam Goodes. And because the world constantly changes, terms of recognition change. Feminism in the 1980s and 1990s, for example, brought about significant changes in the English language, with major implications for how people interacted across gender differences (Davies and Harré, 1990). Who gets to be named as the outsider, as the one to be dispossessed, whose *zersetzung* is to be worked on systematically, changes frequently.

In the USA it is refugees from the south, against whom walls must be erected, and the Chinese, who can conveniently be blamed for the coronavirus pandemic. In Australia, currently, it is refugees who come by boat and are trapped on Manus and Nauru (Boochani, 2018; Davies, 2018). Those in power, such as the Australian prime minister and the home affairs minister, engage in their own identity projects, which are bolstered by dispossession/dis-recognition of those people they can hold outside or in a state of abjection. They claim moral superiority in the "defence of the nation" against those dangerous outsiders whom they refer to as rapists and murderers, and never as humans who have suffered intolerably in their homelands, and who go on suffering at the hands of a government devoid of sympathy. Life's energy has run out for many dispossessed refugees, many of whom have ended their lives in the face of their despair.

There have been large social movements that collectively attempt to let go of past collective acts of dis-recognition: the truth and reconciliation process in South Africa; and in Australia, the *Uluru statement from the heart* (Referendum Council, 2017); both taking enormous generosity of spirit from those who have been badly hurt; both opening those who initiate those movements toward reconciliation to further wilfully cruel acts of dispossession from those who refuse to, or are unable to, recognise the harm they have done and are going on doing.

Attempts at reconciliation can be taken as a chance by perpetrators to open old wounds in the other, with misrepresentations of the truth, and a refusal to admit wrongdoing. The demand that one admits to having done so much violence to the other, against whom or above whom one's identity is formed, turns out to be more than most normalised identities can bear. The court hearing with Superintendent Thomas demonstrated that dynamic. The moral imperatives of one's own safe sense of possession (the first component) may not allow admission of one's own or one's group's acts of dispossession, especially when they are monstrous and inhumane. Of the Truth and Reconciliation Commission, Bishop Tutu observed sorrowfully: "We have all experienced how much better we feel after apologies are made and accepted, but even still it is so hard for us to say that we are sorry" (Tutu, 2004).

Dispossession/dis-recognition, in this analysis, involves speaking to or of a subject in a way that mobilises a different or contrary belief system from the one that gives that subject life. As such it denies their ongoing emergence. This is not just to say something untrue about someone, but to deny their belonging, their knowing in being, and thus the *conditions* of their ongoing emergence.

The treatment of refugees on Manus Island was documented in secret by Boochani (2018), who wrote his account in a series of text messages on his phone. The treatment was characterised by sustained strategies intended to de-humanise them. They were given numbers instead of names on arrival, strip-searched when they quite evidently had no possessions to hide after weeks on their dangerous, life-threatening sea voyages. They were given deliberately ridiculous, humiliating, ill-fitting clothes to wear, then caged indefinitely. De-humanising strategies were deployed night and day, year after year. Not least of those dehumanising strategies was the way they were placed in indefinite detention, having committed no crime, and having no possible means to challenge their detention in court.

Creative-relationality – or response-ability

The third component of recognition, creative-relationality, is where the new and different is celebrated. The first component, possession, cannot thrive without some degree of creative emergence of the new. Yet the impulse to close down the creative emergence of the new is strong. That closing down can be a response of one to another, and it can be systemic, and most likely both. The continuity of life, its capacity to endure, depends not only on normative reiterations, but on the creative acts that open up difference, differenciation, and the creative evolution of the new (Bergson, 1998).

This third component of recognition, creative-relationality arises from our response-ability. In contrast to the first and second components of recognition, this third component is recognition of and response to the grace and vitality in difference, in creative deviations from the known forms by which we are possessed. This third component is akin to Deleuze's *encounters*, or Barad's *intra-actions,* in both of which each participant, human and more-than-human, affects and is affected by the other, such that the world they are of is no longer predictably the same – and nor are they whatever it was they were before, though the shift might be minute. The assemblage shifts, the world shifts, most often in minute creative mo(ve)ments of being.

These movements are intrinsic to the world's liveliness: "There is a vitality to intra-activity, a liveliness, not in the sense of a new form of vitalism, but rather in terms of a *new sense of aliveness*. The world's effervescence, its exuberant creativeness can never be contained or suspended" (Barad, 2007: 234–235; my emphasis).

(Ah, Karen, but it can, it can. The world's aliveness, perhaps, can never be contained or suspended, but for some dispossessed beings, whose life is contained or suspended, the capacity for aliveness can be exhausted; life can lose its capacity or will to sustain itself.)

The entangled interdependence of the three components

The three components of recognition do not exist in isolation from one another; they are intimately entangled, they even depend on each other; the first gives us a (potentially) safe plot of land, the second closes that land in, defending and reinforcing it, drawing boundaries around it and defining normativity in opposition to the outside, while the third expands the safe plot of land and gives it its ongoing vitality. Through the first and second, we come to know "who we are" and "who they are". Their clichés demand little thought, and their actions are justified through one or another ascendant moral framework or assemblage.

But the assemblages which make self and other possible are only one part of human/animal/earthly existence. We also *exceed* ourselves in lines of ascent (Bergson, 1998) and lines of flight (Deleuze and Guattari, 1987). Normativity and creative excess do not function as a binary – one *or* the other, but as one *and* the other, both integral to the more-than-human condition. The functioning life-world has within it a countertendency to the reiterated stability of the normalised world: a "creative spontaneity, and organized function. Always both, in a complexity of mutual imbrication … Functional adaptation is only half the story. The other half is spontaneous and creative" (Massumi, 2015: 13).

Creative spontaneity, or what Massumi calls supernormality, can be thought of as excess, in which the subject (whether human, animal or earth) goes beyond themselves – becoming more-than-normal "in a passionate flash of supernormal becoming" (Massumi, 2015: 14). To recognise such a flash of supernormal becoming, to be affected by it, is to enter into the unexpected movement beyond the already known. That flash of becoming may be so small as to go unrecognised:

> supernormal becoming is a "minimal activity" of life's exceeding itself. It is modest, to the point of imperceptibility. In the nest or in writing, it is a modest gesture, vanishing even, no more than a flash. Yet vital. Potentially of vital importance. Because it may resonate and amplify and shake life's regularities to their object-oriented foundations.
>
> (Massumi, 2015: 14)

And it may be vast, changing everything, like a locust plague, or like the Spanish 'flu that from 1918 to 1920 infected a third of the world's population, or like the current coronavirus pandemic.

We share with other forms of life, it seems, the passion or desire to exceed, and a tendency towards expansion even though that excess is sometimes dangerous, and may lead to collective self-destruction.

The Holly (or Holm) Oak

In the encounter that follows I stretch the concept of recognition as creative-relationality to include the world's matter – to plants, and organic and inorganic matter, and I stretch my intuitive grasp of the other, in search of a sympathetic relationality – towards a mutual more-than-human recognition. In contemplating the ethics of recognition – of what is made to matter and how it is made to matter – I trouble the assumption that humans are exclusive and ascendant in the world's mattering.

To give up that ascendant positioning, Barad explains, requires that we give up on the binary separation between ontology and epistemology:

> The separation of epistemology from ontology is a reverberation of a metaphysics that assumes an inherent difference between human and nonhuman, subject and object, mind and body, matter and discourse. Onto-epistemology – the study of practices of *knowing in being* – is probably a better way to think about the kind of understandings that we need to come to terms with how specific intra-actions matter.
>
> (Barad, 2007: 185; emphasis added)

Barad makes a strong case for including the nonhuman in our thinking about the ways in which our intra-actions matter:

> The inanimate is always being shoved to the side, as if it is too far removed from the human to matter, but that which we call inanimate is still very much bodily and lively. It may seem perverse, unimportant, or meaningless, to attribute memory to an inanimate happening, but that speaks of a failure of imagination that gets stuck at the threshold at one of the most stubborn of all dualisms – the animate/inanimate dualism – that stops animacy cold in its tracks, leaving rocks, molecules, particles, and other inorganic entities on the

other side of death, on the side of those who are denied even the ability to die, despite the fact that particles have finite lifetimes.

(Barad, 2012: 21)

When I first walked under the Holly Oak in the Botanic Garden, its palpable, vibrating energy took me by surprise. My body hummed with the force of it. In my astonishment I experimented with walking in and out of the energy the tree seemed to be generating. It was there, again, below the wide-spreading branches, each time I stepped under them. I didn't have any language with which to make sense of this astonishing encounter with the tree – just as I had found myself without words to make sense of my encounter with the pond just 100 metres away in the same gardens (see Chapter 2).

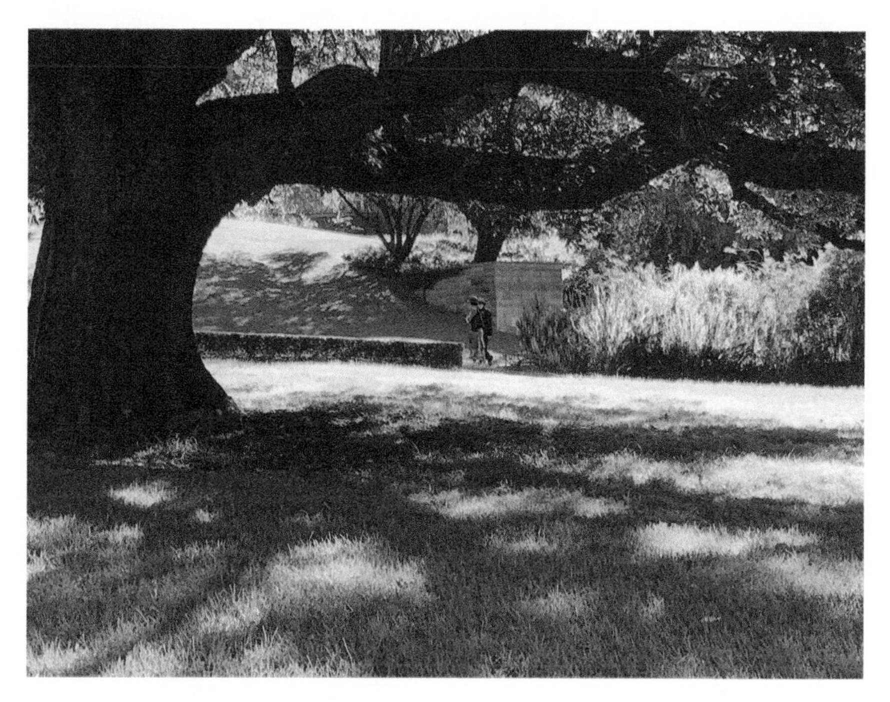

FIGURE 7.1 Holly Oak.
The Royal Botanic Garden, Sydney. Photograph by Bronwyn Davies, 2020.

To begin with, I walked around its trunk and paced out the length of its enormous branches, which reach out horizontally for at least 20 metres on each side. I marvelled at this feat of engineering. I came in close and ran my hands over the rough bark. I felt curiously safe, and I wondered who else the tree might be protecting. In the bark I discovered the exquisite, fine silk webs of tiny spiders who find safe harbour there, their webs like fine silk cloth.

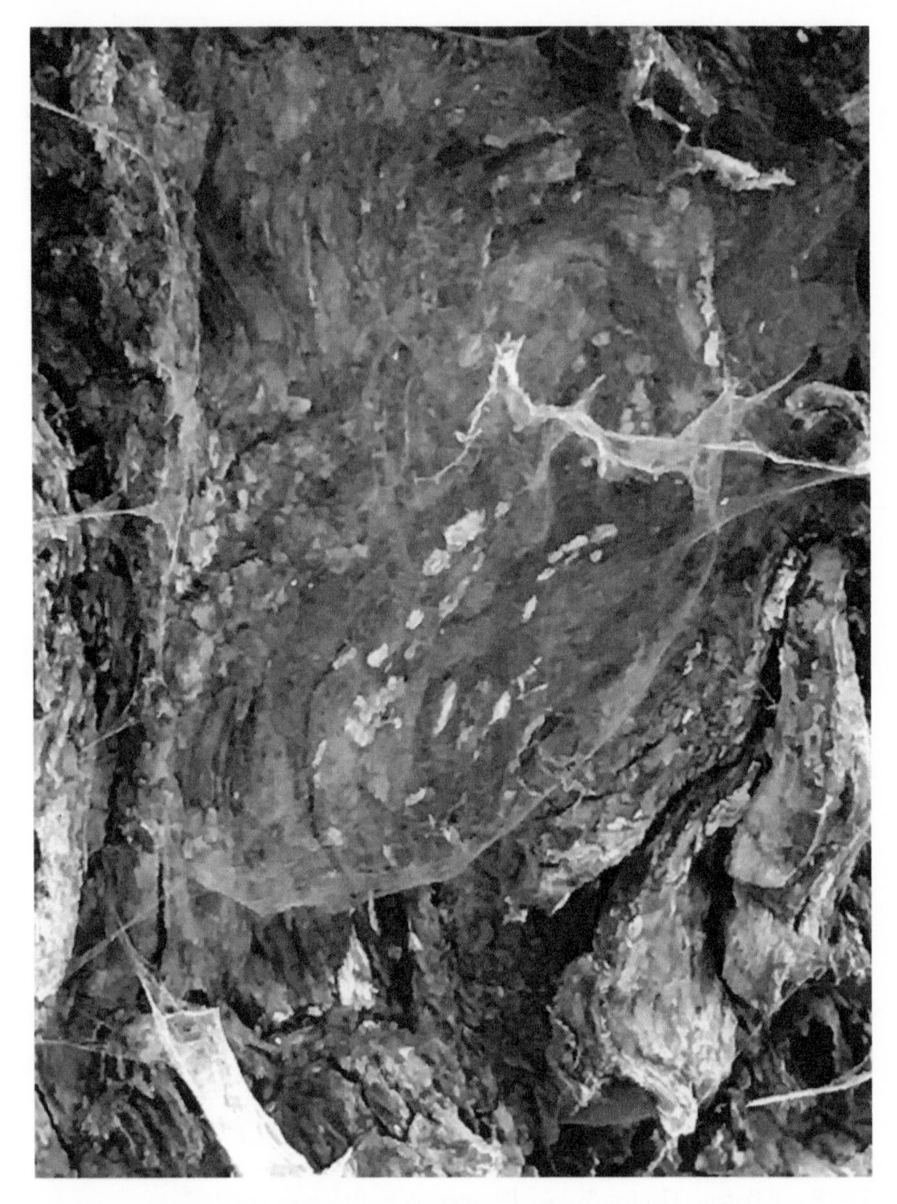

FIGURE 7.2 Spiders' silk cloth.
The Royal Botanic Garden, Sydney. Photograph by Bronwyn Davies, 2019.

On subsequent visits to the Garden I felt myself pulled toward the Holly Oak. Once, when I turned away too soon, I felt a sharp tug pulling me back.

What on earth was going on, I asked myself. How could I learn to read the tree's energy, its thing-power, without anthropomorphising it? To anthropomorphise, as Shaviro (2015) points out, is to assume that all sentience is of the same kind that humans experience with their language-dominated minds. It is to assume, further, that meaningful liveliness, and sympathy, can only take human form.

I wrote in my diary:

I have been visiting the tree most days. I read about Holly Oaks between visits, and discovered that my tree's ancestors came from Europe, just as my own ancestors had (Davies, 2019). Drori wrote of the Holly Oak: "A grand and solid tree with a huge head of densely leafy branches, its charcoal grey bark is broken into small, irregular plates. Its oval leaves resemble those of holly … unusually for an oak it is evergreen; old leaves fall about two years after new ones emerge" (2018: 48). Drori goes on to describe how the Holly Oak provides a small harvest of acorns each year, so the squirrel population is supported; then every few years, all the Holly Oaks in the neighbourhood synchronise to produce a bumper harvest, with far more acorns than the squirrels can eat. It is out of that bumper harvest that acorns can germinate, and new trees grow. But here in the Gardens my Holly Oak is without Holly Oak neighbours, and there are no squirrels.

After weeks of wondering, I finally stopped puzzling. I lay down on the grass under the Holly Oak's branches and gazed up through its leaves and branches to the sky, feeling the dappled sunlight warm on my skin. A soft breeze rippled through the leaves above. Peace descended on me. I heard the songs of the birds, and I fell asleep, embraced within the tree's calm energy, enfolded. I settled, on each subsequent visit, into a sense of belonging with the tree, in an "immediate possession of life qualities *by each other*" (Massumi, 2015: 10–11): "It is this immediate qualitative linkage that constitutes the real conditions of emergence of a subject of experience" (Massumi, 2015: 11). It seemed I had found the passage between us, that enfolded us – that enabled us to engage in an emergent, sympathetic recognition.

Weeks passed. Then:

A few days ago, just before a difficult journey, I was lying under my Holly Oak, resting, as I've taken to doing mid-way on my walk. As I looked up through the branches, I became quite anxious at the thought that one particular branch would fall on me and kill me. I got up from where I was lying, and had lain many times before, and addressed the tree in my mind with a tinge of anger: "So, you would kill me? Why?" My beautiful tree now seemed potentially malevolent and I felt afraid. But the imagined answer came back, that if the branch were to hit me, it would not be deliberate. The fall would be an effect of its extraordinarily long, knotted branches and its age.

So I went to the east side of the tree, outside the circumference of its branches, and lay down again in its shade. No longer so calm. I thought of all the old clichéd humanistic explanations for my sudden fear of the branch falling, my immanent journey, among others. There was nothing about the look of the branch that suggested it was dead or rotten. I was mad, I told myself, to think the tree was communicating with me, warning me of an impending break.

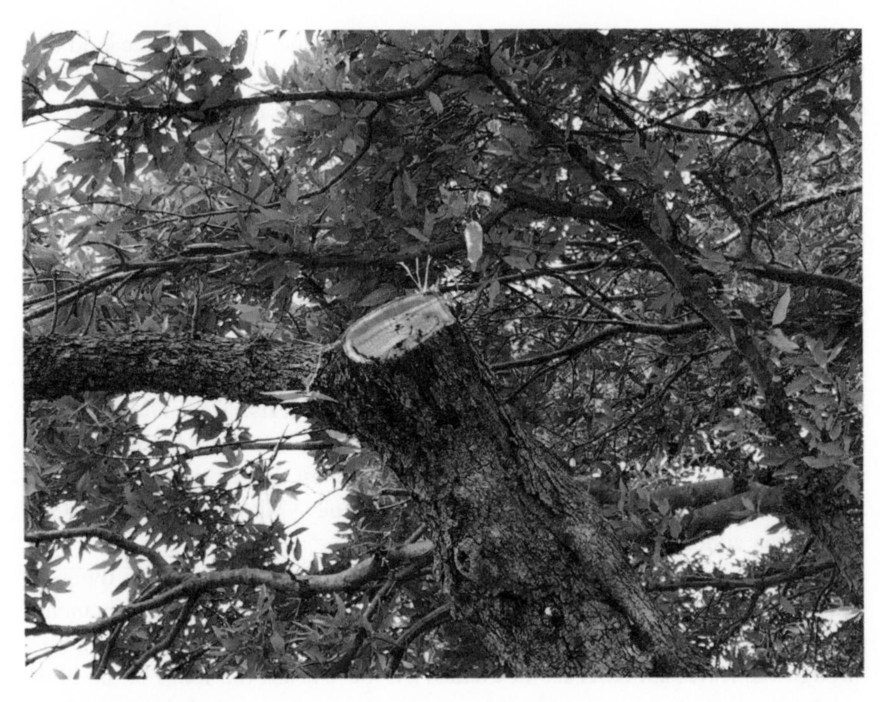

FIGURE 7.3 Stump.
The Royal Botanic Garden, Sydney. Photograph by Bronwyn Davies, 2019.

Today, back from my trip, I went to see if the branch had fallen... I had had vivid images of it falling while I was away. And, sure enough, the potentially offending branch was gone, and in its place fresh saw marks. The gardeners had already tidied up the break.

I lay for a little while in my old spot, looking up at the sawn-off stump, but my old total ease could not, just yet, be recovered.

My capacity to relate to the Holly Oak in the beginning was circumscribed by elements of the first component of recognition, satisfying my romantic longing for the embrace of a protective other. In that sense I effectively narrowed down what it was possible for me to recognise, and become attached to, in the tree. The falling branch brought me, with a jolt, to the realisation that I had more work to do in opening my mind to the possibilities of what this complex encounter with the tree might hold – something far outside what I already took myself to know, lying outside my intuitive capacities, demanding of me that I move further toward the tree, in search of sympathetic relationality. Sympathy must reach through intuition toward a reality outside itself, calling on a greater capacity to engage in emergent listening, opening oneself to the not yet known of the other.

Through reading Powers' (2018) book *The Overstory*, I realise I have been underestimating the capacity of my tree to connect with other trees through its roots. It is not the solitary stranger I have been imagining, but part of a much bigger organism, roots stretched out to other trees, and perhaps not only to other Holly Oaks. In Deleuze's book on Spinoza he observes that commonality between subjects "exists through actions rather than identities or taxonomical classifications" (Stark, 2017: 72). The stronger trees in these vast organisms, I learned, support the weaker trees through these root connections.

I've been thinking about the tree's outstretched branches – not just the extraordinary engineering feat they have engaged in. Now I'm wondering what the branches are reaching toward. What desire led them to stretch so far, not smoothly in one line or gesture, but with knotted joints out of which the next surge outward grows. The tree reaches out again and again. Who or what does it reach out towards? Is it actually as alone as I thought? Bennett says nature "is a place wherein bodies strive to enhance their power of activity by forging alliances with other bodies in their vicinity" (2004: 353).

What other trees and what other beings does it communicate with via its emissions from leaves and bark? What roots does it connect with under the earth? What fungi, what life under the earth does it connect with?

At first I thought its roots might connect with the one other Holly Oak that I had only just discovered – not realising that it might also connect with other trees, not abjecting them because they are categorised by humans as different and unchangeable. The root connections would mean the tree is far from being a solitary subject. Perhaps the reach of its branches echoes the reach of its roots. What other trees does it connect with and lend its strength to?

Lying now under the tree and feeling its vibrations, I realised, before drifting off to sleep, that the vibrations come not just from trunk, branches and leaves, but also from the roots' and the trees' interconnectivity. I found myself in awe of that vastness, and embarrassed at the limited intuition and limiting normativities that had allowed me to see my tree as if it were alone.

As I walked away this time, leaving that vast interconnected life-form behind, I realised for the first time that my mobility was a disadvantage, blinding me to my interconnectivity with the earth and its multiple interconnected beings/becomings. My mobility has made it much easier for capitalist systems to individualise and thus territorialise me, separating me from others. Unlike the Holly Oak, I must connect over and over again, and that makes me dependent on acts of recognition, and always vulnerable to dis-recognition and dispossession.

When I lie under the tree and fall asleep, I exist in peaceful commonality with the immense system of which the tree is a part. Other commonalities I cannot take for granted.

I only discovered the second Holly Oak recently. Its energy is entirely different from *my* Holly Oak. It does not feel safe or welcoming. It actually seems a little mad, as if it's not inter-connected, but intent on becoming a total system entire unto itself.

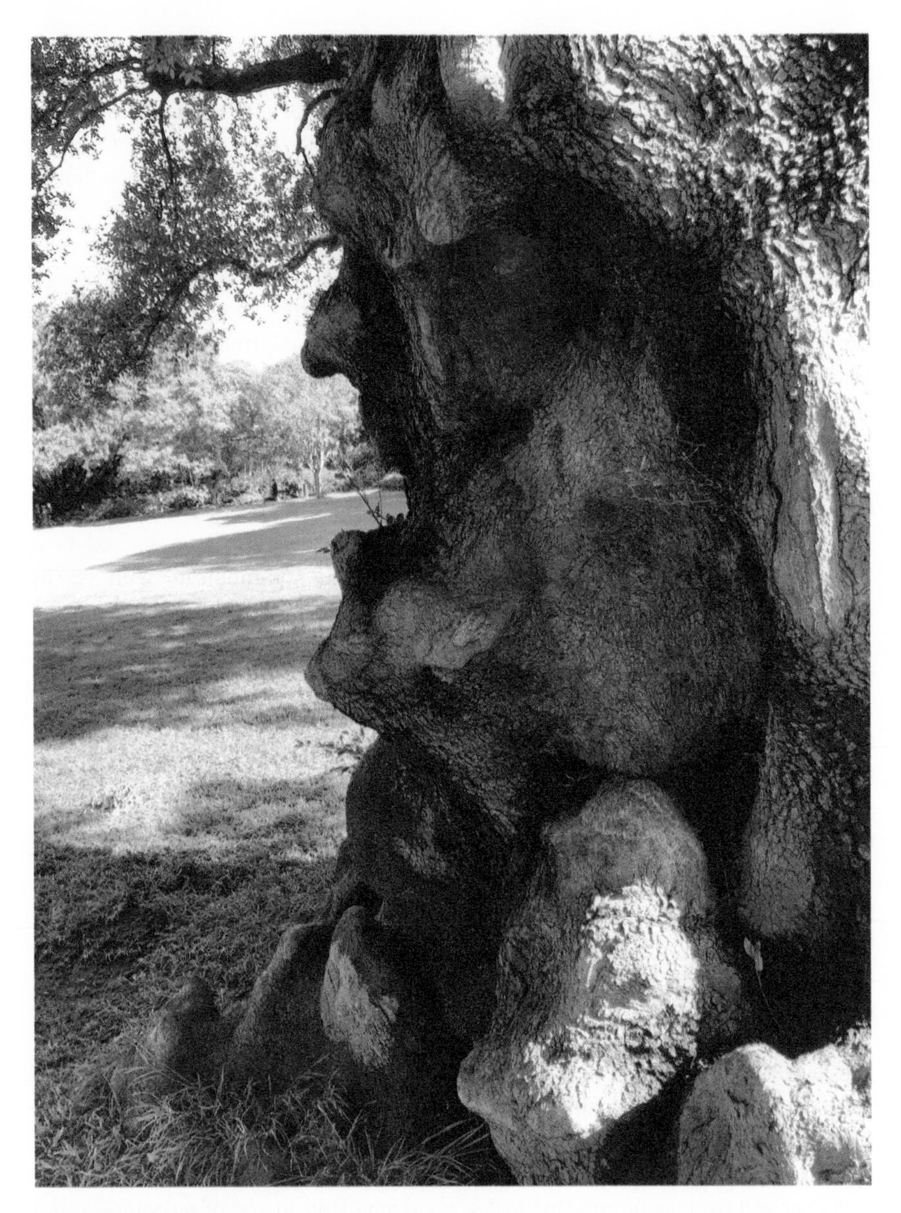

FIGURE 7.4 Mad Oak.
The Royal Botanic Garden, Sydney. Photograph by Bronwyn Davies, 2019.

It is twisted and contorted and bulbous. One of its profiles resembles a face screaming. Its branches reach up more than out, though there is no competition around it for light. It has formed a stagnant pool in its trunk where mosquitoes breed, and its bumps and hollows act as a nursery to shelter acorns that have attempted to sprout out of the way of the Garden's mowers. I am filled with sadness when I stand near its trunk. It belongs in a story of fairies and goblins, of an earth with unfathomable powers. I find myself unable to offer it recognition, since I cannot bear its sadness and isolation.

I am, of course, not proud of that failure.

And so...

> [*We*] *are iteratively reconfigured through each intra-action, thereby making it impossible to differentiate in any absolute sense between creation and renewal, beginning and returning, continuity and discontinuity, here and there, past and future.* .
>
> (Barad, 2007: ix; emphasis added)

To *recognise* the accomplishment of going beyond the already known, when such exceeding often goes unnoticed, and when it may be rejected as inappropriate or wrong, heightens the moment of excess by opening up the life-flow in between. It is that opening up of the flow in-between, in response to a moment of grace – or excess – that gifts me, as witness, with sympathetic becoming, and as such expands my more-than-human life-fullness, passion and desire.

> What we have with the supernormal is a force that pulls forward from ahead, and does so qualitatively: an attractive force. Supernormality is an attractor that draws behaviour in its direction, following its own tendency, not in conformity but deformedly and, surpassing normality, without common measure. Supernormality is not a force of impulsion or compulsion, but *affective propulsion*.
>
> (Massumi, 2015: 9)

And perhaps that is a better way of thinking about my Holly Oak – its powers of affective propulsion, to which I could not help but respond, enabled me to issue forth, expanding in the encounter in ways I could barely comprehend.

Writing, for me, is where my deformational excess is most likely to take place – at least as I am aware of it. This chapter pulled me toward itself, just as the Holly Oak does, offering me a knowing in being beyond the already known – intensifying the experience of life itself, of being in the moment, fully alive. Supernormality has an intensification effect; it is deformational. It may be difficult to grasp. But I know now why those tears come to my eyes when I witness an act of creative-relational recognition, connecting me in that moment to the life-fullness and danger of the deformational line of flight. And I know more vividly than when I set out on this deformational writing, the horror of the act of dispossession, both as I am on the receiving end of it and as I witness it multiplying globally.

Emergent becoming, in its *relationality*, is vulnerable to the way utterances can shift the subject from one assemblage to another, from an assemblage where the subject is creatively flourishing, capable of improvisations that enliven, giving rise to creative evolution or involution and to moments of grace, to one where life-fullness is stifled or even stamped out. Dispossession/dis-recognition repositions the other as at fault, negating their right to a place in a moral/normative order with-in which life can flourish. We each need reiterated, normalised knowing in being, and cannot live without it. We may engage in acts of dis-recognition in support of it. And we each have within us the power to exceed, and to enable those we are becoming-with to evolve, to be life-full, to be more-than-human.

References

Barad, K. 2007. *Meeting the Universe Halfway*. Durham, NC/London: Duke University Press.

Barad, K. 2012. Intra-active entanglements – an interview with Karen Barad. *Kvinder, Køn & Forskning, Gender and Research* 1-2, 10–23.

Barad, K. 2014. Diffracting diffraction: Cutting together-apart. *Parallax*, 20(3), 168–187.

Bennett, J. 2004. The force of things: Steps toward an ecology of matter. *Political Theory*, 32(3), 347–372.

Bergson, H. 1998. *Creative Evolution*. Mineola, NY: Dover Publications Inc.

Boochani, B. 2018. *No Friend but the Mountains* (trans. O. Tofighian). Sydney: Pan Macmillan Australia.

Butler, J. 1997. *The Psychic Life of Power*. Stanford, CA : Stanford University Press.

Davies, B. 2018. Encounters with difference and the entangled enlivening of being. *Departures in Critical Qualitative Research*, 7(4), 1–19.

Davies, B. 2019. *New Lives in an Old Land. Re-turning to the Colonisation of New South Wales through Stories of my Parents and their Ancestors*. Sydney, NSW: Ornythorhynchus Paradoxus Books.

Davies, B. and Harré, R. 1990. Positioning: The discursive production of selves. *Journal for the Theory of Social Behaviour*, 20(1), 43–63.

Deleuze, G. 1994. *Difference and Repetition* (trans. P. Patton). New York: Columbia University Press.

Deleuze, G. 2000. *Proust and Signs. The Complete Text* (trans. R. Howard). Minneapolis, MN: University of Minnesota Press.

Deleuze, G. 2004. *Difference and Repetition*, (trans. P. Patton). London: Continuum.

Deleuze, G. and Guattari, F. 1987. *A Thousand Plateaus. Capitalism and Schizophrenia*, (trans. B. Massumi). Minneapolis, MN: University of Minnesota Press.

Deleuze, G. and Parnet, C. 2007. *Dialogues 11, Revised Edition* (trans. H. Tomlinson and B. Habberjam). New York: Columbia University Press.

Doerr, A. 2007. *Four Seasons in Rome*. London: 4th Estate.

Drori, J. 2018. *Around the World in 80 Trees* (illus. L. Clerc). London: Laurence King Publishing.

Funder, A. 2019–20. Stasiland Now. *The Monthly. Summer Edition*. December to January, 24–38.

Grant, S. 2019. *The Australian Dream* (movie, director Daniel Gordon). Sydney: Madman Films.

Grosz, E. 2001. *Architecture from the Outside*. Cambridge, MA: MIT Press.

Haraway, D. J. 2016. *Staying with the trouble. Making kin in the Chthulucene*. Durham, NC/London: Duke University Press.

Harris, A. M., Holman Jones, S. and Wyatt, J. 2019. Moving, Shaking and Tracking: Micro-Making in Video, Performance and Poetry. *Mai: Feminism & Visual Culture*, 15 May, np.

Hooper, C. 2019–20. Remember her name. The death of Tanya Day. *The Monthly. Summer Edition*, December to January, 60–64.

Lapoujade, D. 2019. Intuition and sympathy in Bergson. *Eidos*, no. 9, np. http://rcientificas.uninorte.edu.co/index.php/eidos/article/viewArticle/1428 Accessed 9-9-19.

Massumi, B. 2015. The supernormal animal. In R. Grusin (ed.), *The Nonhuman Turn*. Minneapolis, MN: University of Minnesota Press, 1–17.

Nancy, J.-L. 2007. *The Creation of the World or Globalization*, (trans. F. Raffoul and D. Pettigrew). Albany, NY: State University of New York Press.

Nancy, J.-L. 2017. *The Possibility of a World. Conversations with Pierre-Philippe Jandin*, (trans. T. Holloway and F. Méchain). New York: Fordham University Press.

Powers, R. 2018. *The Overstory: A Novel*. New York: W. W. Norton and Company.

Referendum Council, 2017. *Uluru statement from the heart*. Referendumcouncil.org.au/.../Uluru_Statement_From_The_Heart_o.pdf.

Shaviro, S. 2015. Consequences of panpsychism. In R. Grusin (ed.), *The Nonhuman Turn*. Minneapolis, MN: University of Minnesota Press, 19–44.

Shildrick, M. 2002. *Embodying the Monster: Encounters with the Vulnerable Self*. London: SAGE.

Stark, H. 2017. *Feminist Theory after Deleuze*. London: Bloomsbury Academic.

Tutu, D, 2004. Truth and Reconciliation. *Greater Good Magazine*, 1 Sept, np.

Wyatt, J. 2019. *Therapy, Stand-up, and the Gesture of Writing*. New York: Routledge.

8

INTUITION AND THE FLOW IN BETWEEN ONE AND ANOTHER

> In which I focus on encounters between my own life as a researcher, and the life of another. I look at the liveliness of language in those encounters, those acts of recognition, or dis-recognition, and I contemplate some of the bad habits that Cartesian humanism and "scientific method" can lead us into. I draw on stories from my book New Lives in an Old Land and I extend my analysis of those stories, drawing on art, and on the concepts of duration and intuition.

> *intuition is the art – the manner – in which the very conditions of experience are felt … intuition activates the proposition at the heart of the as yet unthought.*
>
> (Manning, 2015: 45; emphasis added)

In Chapter 1, I explored the ways in which life emerges out of the entangled dynamics of social, material and semiotic flows and forces. In the intervening chapters I have re-turned to life's capacity to endure, where "duration means invention, the creation of forms, the continual elaboration of the absolutely new" (Bergson, 1998: 11). In this chapter I focus on the singular existence of "a life", and on encounters between one life and another. New materialisms focus on the flow in between one and another, and on life's multiplicative capacity, and I contemplate the way a life can lose sight of passion, of intensity and of the singularity of embodied existence. Wyatt writes:

> However inadequate, however provisional, however misleading, we can and we must claim the possibility of singularity; we can and must aspire to, and work at, creating such singularity through writing …When I talk about singularity I am talking here of the "singular existent" of Nancy, which "may be singular-plural or something else entirely, outside of the order of the calculable".
>
> (Wyatt, 2019: 127, citing Nancy, 2000)

Allowing singular voices to emerge from collective assemblages, is not to re-evoke "the fixed, centred, bounded, unitary, denominative subject," Wyatt argues, but rather "something like Caverero's *unique existent* ... needing the other's recognition and therefore always vulnerable, always incomplete. It is characterized by desire, she says, and in particular the desire for narration by the other" (Wyatt, 2019: 129–30). The stories through which we make life make sense and through which we take up our own singularity – our own extraordinariness – make life possible, even while potentially containing and constraining it.

I re-turned in my last book (2019) to the lives of my ancestors. I re-turn again here to three of those lives: to my great-great-uncle Thomas, to my great-great-grandmother, Mary Nivison, and my mother Norma.

In that re-turning I further open up the encounter with each of them in order to stretch my engagement with the singularity and the multiplicative force of their lives as I animate them in my writing. As I do so I must remember to remain vigilant about the work that my modes of knowledge-making are doing. Our habitual categorisations, for example, limit our capacity to see the unexpected and our capacity to be open to what we don't yet know. As Bergson (1998: x) observes of the work of scientists: "In vain we force the living into this or that one of our molds. All the molds crack. They are too narrow, above all too rigid for what we try to put into them." The work of new materialist research, then, involves us in detecting and escaping those limiting habits of categorisation, and in opening up new possibilities of questioning, and of engaging.

Bergson stresses the vital link between studying life, and studying the process of knowledge-making itself: "It is necessary that these two inquiries, theory of knowledge and theories of life, should join each other, and, by a circular process, push each other on unceasingly" (Bergson, 1998: xiii). Human subjects, far from being finite, are in a constant state of change: "there is no feeling, no idea, no volition which is not undergoing change every moment" (Bergson, 1998: 1), and "for a conscious being, to exist is to change, to change is to mature, to mature is to go on creating oneself endlessly" (Bergson, 1998: 7). And that endless creation is always relational. Like the organs of the body, which work in relation to each other, and depend on each other, humans are entangled in interdependent relations with others – human, animal and earth others, with practical and artistic others. In social, material and semiotic flows, life's emergence and endurance is a matter of entanglement:

> The very nature of materiality is an entanglement. Matter itself is always already open to, or rather entangled with, the "Other." The intra-actively emergent "parts" of phenomena are coconstituted. Not only subjects but also objects are permeated through and through with their entangled kin; the other is not only in one's skin, but in one's bones, in one's belly, in one's heart, in one's nucleus, in one's past and future.
>
> (Barad, 2007: 392–393)

What happens, then, in encounters between researchers and the subjects of their inquiries, does not produce a truth that exists independent of the inquiry. The truth lies in the flow in-between, in *what comes alive* in each encounter. That movement in-between, Bergson calls "reciprocal interpenetration" (Bergson, 1998: 178), or *sympathetic communication*, which enables "the expansion of our consciousness" and our "endlessly continued creation" (Bergson: 1998, 177–178). This is akin to the third component of recognition that I explored in Chapter 7.

Sympathetic communication in research encounters depends on the capacity to listen to the not-yet-known. It demands of us that we be open to movement, to the flow of affect, to the unexpected, to new continuities and to discontinuities. Such listening depends on an intensification of the senses, or what Nancy calls "stretching the ears": "an expression that evokes a singular mobility among the sensory apparatuses, of the pinna of the ear – it is an intensification and a concern, a curiosity or anxiety" (Nancy, 2007: 5). To listen to the flow in between one and another depends on the stretching of all the senses; it depends on intuition.

Intuition, Bergson argues, is what enables us to explore life *from within life itself.* This is not an undisciplined floating free of thought, but the setting free of a vital force that enables a rigorous innovative exploration of the question being researched. For Bergson, intuition enables us to go beyond experience "toward the conditions of experience" (Deleuze, 1991: 27).

Getting stuck: Great-great-uncle Thomas

If life gets locked into an unceasing repetition, then intuition, sympathy, creativity and relationality can all be shut down. Institutions that forcibly shut down change, and foreclose all possibility of creative evolution, can literally break lives. In Australian offshore detention centres, refugees are held indefinitely and without trial for years on end. One of the most chilling cruelties in those centres is the forbidding of play. "No games" the guards scream, when detainees invent a way to play a board game. "No games!" No holding on to life's capacity to create, to set things in motion, to affirm life when stuck in indefinite detention; this is an institutional cruelty that is systematically intent on your *Zersetzung,* your breakdown, decomposition, degradation (Boochani, 2018).

Sometimes creative-relationality is broken, not through such systematic, egregious inhumanity, but through a collective or singular thought that gets caught in a repeating chain, citing and re-citing itself without end. Such recitations may be tied to perceived injustice and loss. They may perpetuate an obsession with particular categories and the perceived borders between self and other. Such endless recitations may put a block on the continuous movement and change that enables life to endure.

Take, for example, the obsession of my great-great-uncle, Thomas Hughes Ford Hughes. Thomas became obsessed with the loss to 'foreigners' of the Davies family's Welsh estate, *Nant Gwylan*:

> Thomas Hughes Forde Hughes … died in Wales on March 8 1914. He had once been a talented and successful young man, but in his 30s he became a recluse, and at the same time accrued vast amounts of property – and mortgages – the prize property being the original *Nant Gwylan*, which had been sold out from under his mother's feet, to "foreigners".
>
> (Davies, 2019: 77)

The newspaper report of his death told the story of his decline:

> *Landowner's Death in the Workhouse (1914)*
>
> *Eccentric Recluse leaves £74,000*
>
> *Mr Thomas Ford Hughes, who died in the Carmarthen Workhouse on March 8, has left estate worth £74,000, and letters of administration have been granted to his sister, Miss Ellen Lloyd Davies of Carmarthen.*
>
> *For many years, Mr Hughes had lived the life of a recluse in a cottage in Carmarthen which no one was allowed to enter. When he became seriously ill, he still refused all help and on March 2 last, the authorities made a forcible entry and removed him to the workhouse.*
>
> *Mr Ford Hughes owned the Aberceri and Nant Gwylan estates in Cardiganshire as well as land in Pembrokeshire. He was born in 1840 and his original name was Davies, but he adopted that of Hughes by deed poll on succeeding to the estate of his maternal uncle.*
>
> *He lived a normal life until he was about thirty years old but then for some unknown reason he became addicted to solitude. He took a cottage in Carmarthen and when he visited his mansions he would hire a carriage and travel at night. After a time, he gave up even these visits and he never left the Carmarthen cottage after 1887.*
>
> *For years no one visited his house except a barber, and when the barber died, Mr Hughes allowed his hair and beard to grow. His meals were sent in from hotels but nobody got further than the door.*
>
> *The grimy windows of the house were familiar to the Carmarthen people for nearly thirty years. The town council often discussed the possibility of the sanitary inspector procuring a warrant to enter but no action was taken as no nuisance could be proved. Two years ago there was a fire at the cottage and persons who saw the interior declare that ashes had accumulated in piles around the fire and that newspapers and books were stacked to the ceiling.*
>
> *When the authorities entered on March 2, the door of the bedroom had to be pushed back inch by inch as the ashes and rubbish were shovelled out.*

The family's fortune, had it remained entailed, would eventually have gone to my father. It had dwindled to almost nothing once the mortgages were paid. What was left went to Thomas's sister, who left it to her servant.

For 30 years of Thomas Hughes Ford Hughes' life, one refrain circled and re-circled, shutting down the possibility of a life; the family estate had been lost to foreigners and must be recovered – over and over again. All else had become irrelevant. When he bought *Nant Gwylan*, he restored it to its former glory, then locked the door and let it go to ruin. A grand piano, which wouldn't fit through the front door, was left to rot outside. He continued to buy more properties, which he let out to tenants who could take care of them. He never cashed their cheques, piling them up for years in the dust and ruins of the cottage he had shut himself into. Through his continual repetition of the same act, buying another property, taking out another mortgage, the past wrong grew larger and larger, taking over his life. The past is not usually so perfectly preserved as it was for Thomas. Bergson observes that "Duration is the continuous progress of the past which gnaws into the future and which swells as it advances. And as the past grows without ceasing, so also there is a limit to its preservation." However perfectly or imperfectly preserved, the past "follows us at every instant; all that we have felt, thought and willed from our earliest infancy is there, leaning over the present which is about to join it, pressing upon the portals of consciousness that would fain leave it outside" (Bergson, 1998: 4–5).

Thomas had grown up in the Victorian 1800s in the bright Welsh sunshine and mists of *Nant Gwylan: Home of the Seagulls*. He had successfully embarked on a military career, serving Queen Victoria's project of expanding British power and God's word throughout the Empire. His place as the eldest son meant he was to inherit *Nant Gwylan* and become, in time, the 'Lord of the Manor'. When *Nant Gwylan* was sold to 'foreigners' his anticipated place in the world was lost. The past life that had promised certainty, gnawed into the future and swallowed it whole. He disappeared inside the loss, and no amount of acquisition, even the acquisition of *Nant Gwylan* itself, could release him from the refrain of that past wrong.

On my first re-turn to Thomas, I struggled to develop a sympathetic relationship with him. Who, after all, wants to own a mad uncle? But mindful of my failure to sympathise with the second Holly Oak (see Chapter 7), I decided to re-turn again. The combination of research and writing about our shared ancestry, combined with new materialist concepts enabled a new flow in between.

Thomas and I were descended from Tudwall Gloff, the fourth, or in some accounts fifth, son of Rhodri Mawr, King of all Wales. Rhodri Mawr married Angharad, Queen of South Wales, and after the death of his father, Rhodri Mawr ruled a united Wales from 844 to 877. That period of 33 years is the only time there has been a king of all Wales. Tudwall Gloff, or Tudwall the Lame, however, was not the son of Queen Angharad. His place among his legitimate brothers was tenuous from the beginning. Then he was wounded at the age of 16 fighting in one of his brother's armies, in one of the many wars defending

Wales against the invading hordes of Danes and of English. Welsh law dictated that lame people could not inherit property, so he was damned twice over, being illegitimate at a time when that mattered, and disinherited by state law, for being lame.

Thomas's obsession with the loss of *Nant Gwylan,* of being dispossessed of his place in it, was a continuation of a story that had begun with Tudwall Gloff.

My life was not impervious to that history. When my parents sold our family's rural Australian home, the home my father had wanted to call *Nant Gwylan*, I was outraged: "Oh, well, that's it then," I said to my poor mother, on the phone, "there's no point in my ever coming home again." I was 20 years old at the time. The house my parents were selling had sheltered and protected me in a way my parents often had not. It provided the space in which my senses, and my sense of myself, my singularities, came into being. It was where I learned to exist. It is still in my skin – in my blood, in my bones, in my imagination. I can still smell it, taste it, hear it, feel it. My material being and the house were entangled with each other – and still are, just as Thomas was entangled with the original *Nant Gwylan*.

Thomas and I, and the two *Nant Gwylans*, were/are/will be of the same matter, continuous with each other, even while separated by vast stretches of time and place. (I continue to call my family home *Nant Gwylan*, as my father wished, though my mother would never agree to it being given that name. It was always referred to as 98).

At the time of writing I am forced into self-isolation for an indefinite period of time as part of the government's response to the coronavirus pandemic. I can see that if this went on long enough, instead of railing against the confinement I would begin to desire it. During my marriage I was cut off from human contact, and the horror of that memory leads me to keep alive my desire to go out. I have created a small artwork for my front door that maintains the illusion that I can always see through it and beyond it.

I found the frame on the footpath, where a couple who were moving to a smaller flat were abandoning their unwanted furniture. I suggested to them they should keep the frame, since it was so beautiful. It used to hold the picture of her daughter she told me, and it came from her home country, New Zealand. But she was ready to let it go. I brought it home and polished it. I had been wanting to make an artwork for my door ever since the shutdown, an artwork that would create the illusion of a window that I could see through. It being a company title building I cannot make actual windows in my door. The original windows over the doors have been boarded over in response to fire safety regulations. The image in my artwork is of a deep blue agapanthus. As the light shifts, I sometimes glimpse the agapanthus, and sometimes a silhouette of myself walking toward me; but mostly I appear to have a window, and that window lifts any feeling of being shut in.

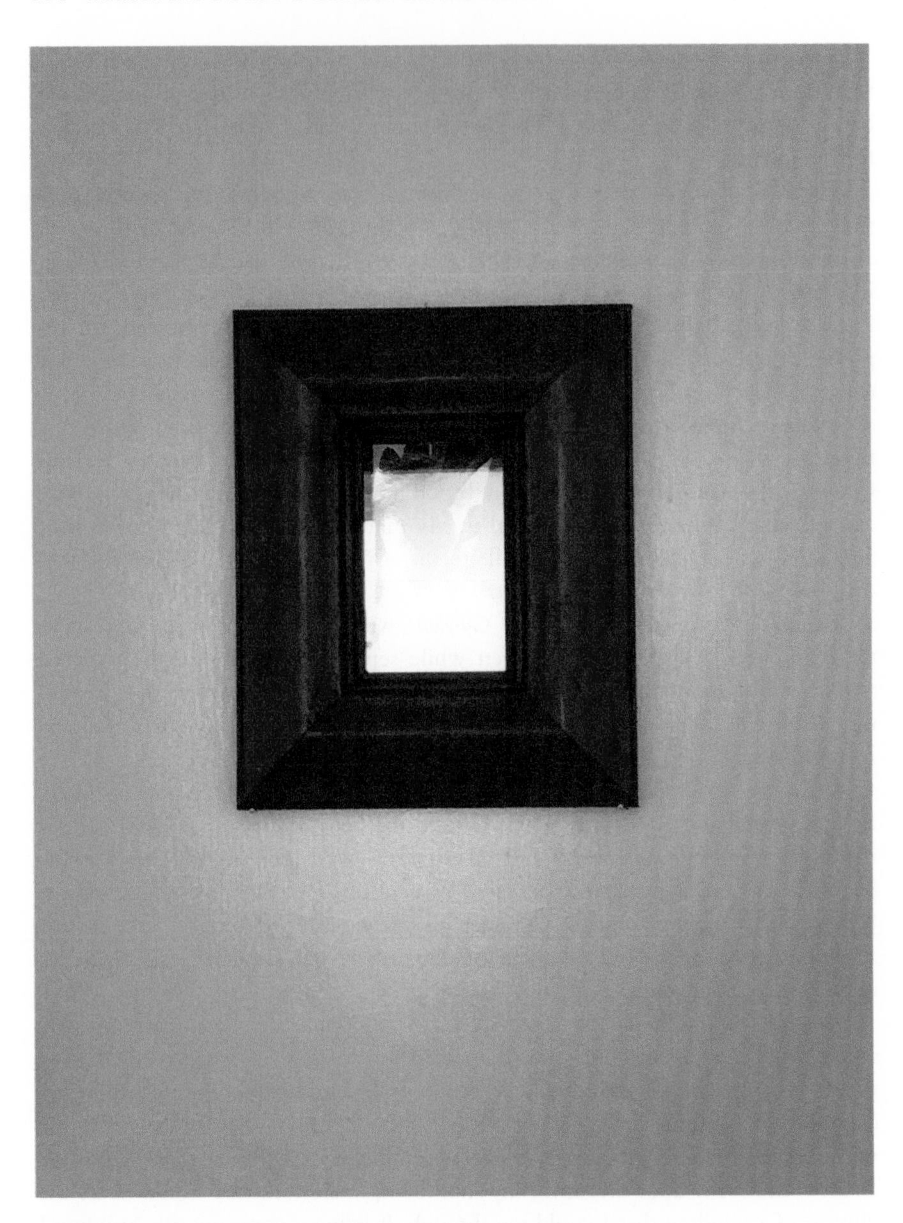

FIGURE 8.1 Bronwyn Davies, A window in my front door. Trompe-l'oeil. Photograph by Bronwyn Davies, 2020.

The bridal veil: My great-great-grandmother Mary

In the ancestral research that formed the possibility of a connection with Thomas, I imagined myself as an orb-weaver spider. I wrote: "I discovered it takes both stillness and perseverance, and many breaks, to be a weaver of entangled family webs. It's to do with the matter and mattering of your own body, your own life, as it is penetrated by, and emergent within the lives of others" (Davies, 2019: xiii). Who anyone is, is not a simple matter of mapping past facts, nor a matter of creating a web made once and for all. Any beginning, Barad (2010: 244) says, like my spider's web, "is always already threaded through with anticipation of where it is going" but unlike the spider's, a family web is searching for a destination it "will never simply reach" and is searching for "a past that has yet to come" (Barad, 2010: 244).

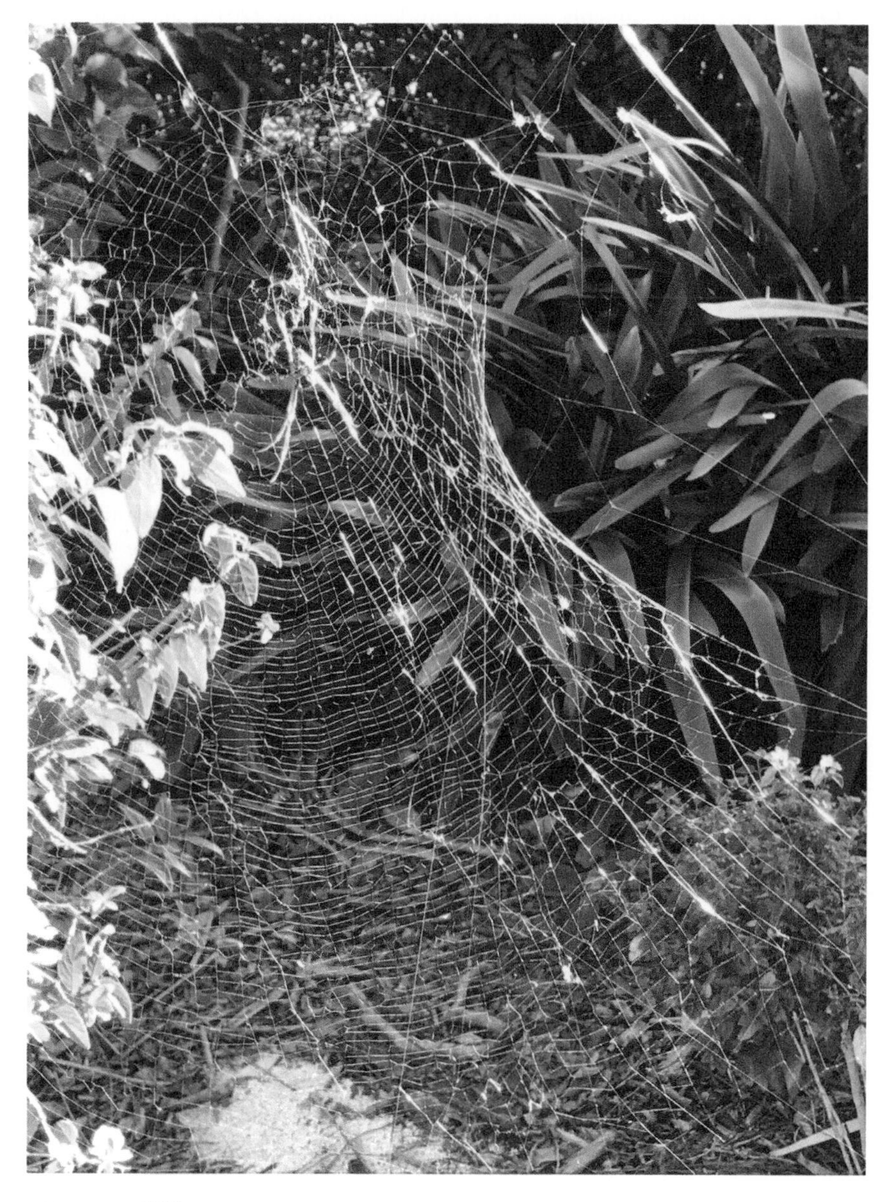

FIGURE 8.2 Web.
The Royal Botanic Garden, Sydney. Photograph by Bronwyn Davies, 2019.

Telling tales of ancestral lives is never a simple matter of discovering what has already been. It is an act of love and of response-ability, but it is also, sometimes, a coming apart and a tearing open – an entanglement in a past that has yet to come: "a repetition, another layer, the return of the same, a catching on something else, an imperceptible difference, a coming apart and ineluctable tearing open" (Deleuze, 1995: 84).

One of the most difficult aspects of undertaking my (2019) ancestral study came with the necessity of reading the accounts of the past written by historians. They had assembled a great deal of useful information relevant to my ancestors' lives that I was dependent on, but the information was accompanied by a peculiar hollowing out of the past, or what Manning calls backgridding. Measurement, or backgridding of the past "'after the fact' tends to deplete the event-time of its middling, deactivating the relational movement that was precisely event-time's force. Backgridded, experience is reconceived in its poorest state: out of movement" (Manning, 2015: 46).

I also found in historians' accounts an obsession with the location of particular objects, such as gravestones, for example, or in the case of Mary, her bridal veil. The historian of the Nivison family was Jillian Oppenheimer, my mother's cousin. In her book *An Australian Clan: The Nivisons of New England* (Oppenheimer and Mitchell, 1989), she wrote about our ancestors, Abraham and Mary Nivison, who migrated from Scotland to the colony of New South Wales in 1839. Mary and Abraham were wed only days before they set sail on their seven-month journey. The family story passed down through the generations was that Mary had worn a veil at the wedding, which had been given to her by a friend who lived in the Manor of the 3rd Duke of Buccleuch, on whose vast estate in the lowlands of Scotland, Mary's and Abraham's families were tenant farmers.

But Jillian could find no veil. If it had been passed down from oldest daughter to oldest daughter, as it was supposed to have been, it should have been possible to find it. When no veil was found, Jillian appealed to class and gender categories for explanation. Since Mary's and Abraham's families were only tenant farmers, she surmised, it was unlikely that the gift had ever been given. Mary, by implication, was a minor fabulist, generating the story of the veil to furnish her new station in life in the colony with a direct, material connection to the rural elite in Scotland.

One of the very few things Jillian wrote about Mary, other than the dates of the births and deaths of her children, and other than the absence of the veil, was that she would have been miserable on the journey to the colony. When I asked Jillian "what is it you know about Mary that you haven't told us, that leads to the conclusion that she was miserable," she looked at me astonished: "She *would have been*! She was pregnant. Those early journeys were horrendous!" So, no evidence from Mary's life that she was inclined toward misery, yet she had been consigned to a backgridded history that assumed she *would have been*. Through such backgridding, women are held in a lesser place. Mary could be relegated to a minor and miserable place in Abraham's story, and in history.

In reading books like Jillian's, I was confronted by the absence of detail about women's lives, and by the absence of the men and the women who had built their houses, tilled their land, taken care of their children, cleaned their houses, and cooked for them. I was further confronted by the absence of the original custodians of the land, who had been displaced by successive waves of British colonists. I found the authoritative and judgemental tone of the scientific/historical method oppressive, and yet, as I struggled to make my own account, I found its language creeping into my own writing, and constricting what it was possible to think. I found myself writing and re-writing, frustrated by the way my own words were drained of life.

To begin my rebellion against the linguistic forms that were invading my writing I made a simple decision to reverse the order of all the couples' names. No longer Abraham and Mary, they were Mary and Abraham. I also weeded out verbs like "would have been". It's surprising how much difference those two small changes made.

In the absence of surviving documentation from Mary's life, I read about the place-time she had grown up in, and about Presbyterianism, as it was at the time. I read, as well, whatever I could find of first-hand accounts of rural life in Scotland in the early 1800s, which included an astonishing number of pregnancies out of wedlock, with the expectant mothers routinely taking their lovers to court to force them to wed. I read, as well, first-hand accounts of ocean voyages from Britain to the colony in the 1700s and 1800s. I visited art galleries and studied visual images of oceans and ships, and ship's voyages in the mid-1800s.

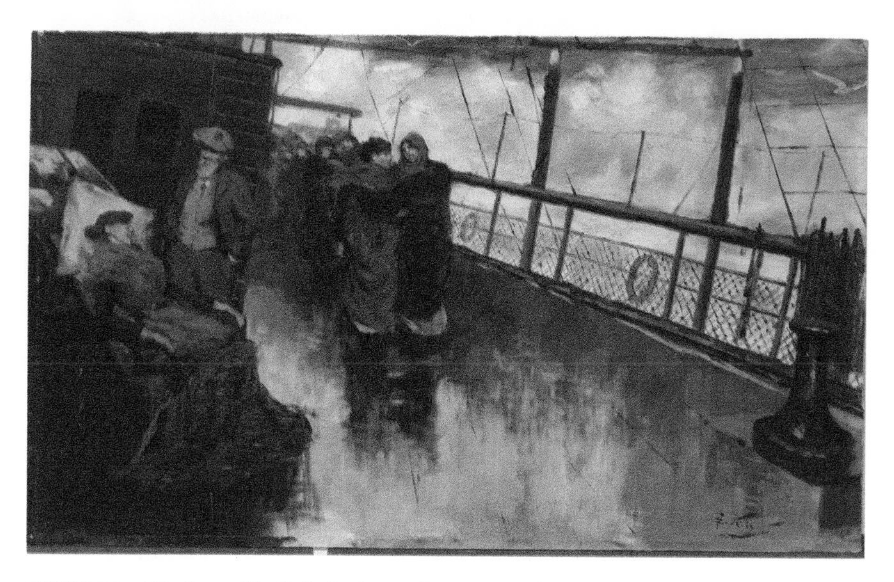

FIGURE 8.3 Girolamo Nerli (Italy; Australia; New Zealand, b. 1860, d. 1926), *The Voyagers* (c. 1890), oil on paperboard, 32.7 × 55 cm.
Art Gallery of New South Wales, Australia, purchased 1952. Photo by AGNSW, Jenni Carter 8688.

This wonderful painting by Girolamo Nerli, *The Voyagers*, enabled me to begin to imagine life on board. I had imagined it as turned outward to the extraordinary vista of the ocean. In Nerli's painting a storm rages at sea; it is lit by the slanting rays of the sun and reflected in the wet deck. But all the passengers are turned in toward each other. The grandeur of the journey takes second place to the intimate flow in between one and another of the human passengers.

I studied, as well, the two remaining photos of Mary, which had been taken when she was much older and ill from the thyroid condition, which she eventually died from, her throat swollen up to the size of a grapefruit. I closely studied the photos of her daughters taken when they were the age Mary was when she had set out on that journey with Abraham in 1839. Jemima, her second daughter, looked most like her.

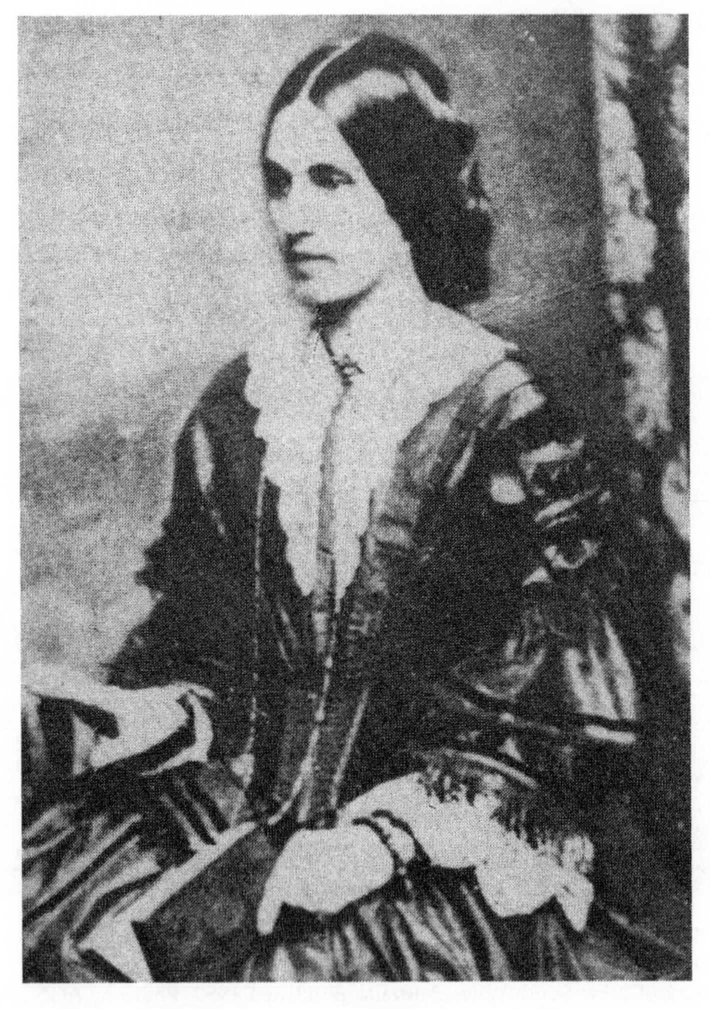

FIGURE 8.4 *Jemima Nivison.*
Photograph from Oppenheimer and Mitchell, *An Australian Clan*, 1989: 59.

My task in writing about Mary was to intuit my way, through my own duration, into Mary's. Citing Deleuze, Manning explains how intuition is vital to such movements in between:

> In its feeling-forth of future potential, intuition draws on time. It touches the sensitive nerve of time. Yet intuition is not duration per se. "Intuition is rather the movement by which we emerge from our own duration, by which we make use of our own duration to affirm and immediately to recognize the existence of other durations" (Deleuze, 1991: 33). Intuition is the relational movement through which the present begins to co-exist with its futurity, with the quality or manner of the not-yet that lurks at the edges of actual experience. This is art: the intuitive potential to activate the future, to make the middling of experience felt where futurity and presence coincide, to invoke the memory not of what was, but of what will be. Art, the memory of the future.
>
> (Manning, 2015: 45–46)

The journey, in 1839, is a work of art yet to emerge through sympathetic listening, or creative-relational recognition; through telling a story which is perhaps the one she would have wished had been told.

Mary and Abraham's journey from Scotland to the colony of New South Wales in 1839 was their honeymoon. Mary had agreed to make that extraordinary seven-month journey across the globe. She may even have been the one who initiated it. She pooled her inheritance with Abraham's to make the journey possible. On board ship they were meeting new people, visiting new places; all their senses were being enlivened in ways they could never have imagined beforehand. They were leaving behind a small community, albeit one that had been through massive changes in their lifetimes, with schools introduced, substantial stone houses built to replace their mud brick cottages, and innovative farming methods brought by the 3rd Duke from Europe where he had travelled with his tutor, the renowned Adam Smith. Mary and Abraham were taking with them the knowledge and the life-forms that they would draw on to re-create a life-sustaining community far from their interdependencies on the Buccleuch estate. The ship's journey was the first place-time of their intimate life together. I wrote, in the first re-turn, of Mary's journey with Abraham:

> [P]erhaps the gift of the veil was real … [If it were, it would open up] a reading of Mary and Abraham in which they are not only sensible, pragmatic Scots, but also romantically entangled; and perhaps, too, it opens the possibility that the Nivisons and Wightmans were sufficiently well-respected by the Duke's family and their immediate circle, to attract such a gift …
>
> [T]he seas in 1839 were alive with multiple life forms …
>
> Did Mary and Abraham look out at these new elements of life on the ocean, or was their gaze turned inward, to life on board the ship, to the people they were travelling with, who were setting out on the same adventure? And in their own cabin were there tender scenes of seduction and pleasurable love-making?
>
> (Davies, 2019: 368–371)

I have imagined that journey as quite different from the backgridded version in which Mary is reduced to someone who is miserable, and whose story need never be told. I cannot, of course, tell where Mary begins and ends, or where Abraham begins and ends, or where I, as writer, begin or end, in this writing of Mary's journey:

> ***1839***
> Snug at last in their cabin
>   she draws the veil over her face
> blushing.   Her beloved,
>   alone and steadfast,
> enduring
>   through all those deaths
>   has found
> a fountain of life in her ...
>   Mary, his graceful doe.
> Tenderly he strokes
>   her quivering flank
>   and draws aside the veil...

A flash of intuition: My mother Norma

Mary was my mother's great-grandmother. She had seven children. I could tell you here the names and dates and places of the birth and death of each of those seven children, and of the 40 grandchildren, and I could thus engage in some mind-numbing backgridding. Much more interesting are "their fluids, their fibers, their continuums and conjunctions of affects, the wind, fine segmentation, microperceptions" (Deleuze and Guattari, 1987: 162). "Becomings, becomings-animal, becomings-molecular" (Deleuze and Guattari, 1987: 162) which I tried to untangle when I wrote about Mary's great-granddaughter, my mother, Norma.

I was startled when an old friend I had not seen for years commented in relation to my ancestral book (2019) that she had enjoyed reading it, but that I had been too hard on my mother. This seemed strange coming from someone who had never met my mother. I protested that if she had known her, she would know that I had been quite generous. But she was adamant. I had been too hard, even harsh. The paragraph she objected to was:

> Norma and Tom didn't marry until 1939. It was a long engagement. Tom's law firm was doing well. He was handsome and charming, and in those early days there was a great deal of laughter and fun – playing tennis and golf, and swimming, and partying. The promise of laughter and wealth. He promised, as well, international travel, a car of her own at a time when only one in ten families owned a car. He would employ a maid to do the housework and to take care of the children. She need never work again. Was she marrying for love as Tim [her sister] had advised? Quite possibly not. The wife he believed was frigid quite simply didn't love him.
>
> (Davies, 2019: 55)

It was this last sentence that my friend especially objected to.

The flash of insight, that my mother hadn't loved my father, had taken me by surprise. You see such flashes in popular detective stories: no one can make sense of all the detail that has been so painstakingly gathered, then, suddenly, the hero/detective has an intuitive flash that causes all the disconnected pieces to fall into place. I was sitting in my favourite coffee shop at the time when my flash of insight happened. I sat staring into space for a long while, absorbing the monstrousness of what I had discovered, and through which the affective flows that made up my family could shift. I groaned internally "Oh, Mum, how could you? How much sadness you brought on us all, how much sadness you brought on yourself and my father."

My mother died in 1994. But her life was not past. The past, as Barad says, is yet to happen. She had loved someone else; I had found evidence of that. But she married someone she could depend on, so she would never be poor, as her family had been poor during the Great Depression in the 1930s. In 1930 she had been put to work as a seamstress in the family of her best, private-school friend. That was a humiliation she never really managed to forget. The traces of the Depression lasted a lifetime.

My friend's challenge to my account raised a question about the flow in between me and my mother. In doing so, it opened the possibility that it could take a different course. But her challenge lingered for some months, with no new course emerging. Then, one day, quite by chance, I found myself staring at the reprint of a painting by John Brack, called *The New House*, that had serendipitously arrived in the mail. I didn't much like the painting, but it kept pulling me toward it. I looked forward to going to the exhibition, but the pandemic arrived, and the gallery closed before the exhibition could be held.

After a while I closed the magazine and filed it away. Yet I felt it pressing so hard on me that I had to get it out again. I had it open, then, next to me, for day after day, not able to access what it seemed so insistently to be telling me. Then suddenly, I had another intuitive flash. What the painting re-opens is the condition of marriage in the 1950s along with the reminder that my task is to open up a movement that goes beyond experience "*toward the conditions of experience*" (Deleuze, 1991: 27; emphasis added). It is obvious, the painting tells me, that it could never have been that simple, that Norma had made a decision to marry my father that was not based on love. I had invoked, implicitly, a causal line running between a decision (including an implied intention to marry for reasons other than love) and our/my unhappiness as children, and even our subsequent failed marriages.

Brack's painting opened up that different course I had been looking for. It transported me into the time and place of my mother's marriage. Brack himself had been a soldier in the Second World War. The bridge in the painting hanging in the new house is one of Van Gogh's many 1888 paintings of Langlois Bridge, a drawbridge, one that had been blown up by the Germans when they were in retreat.

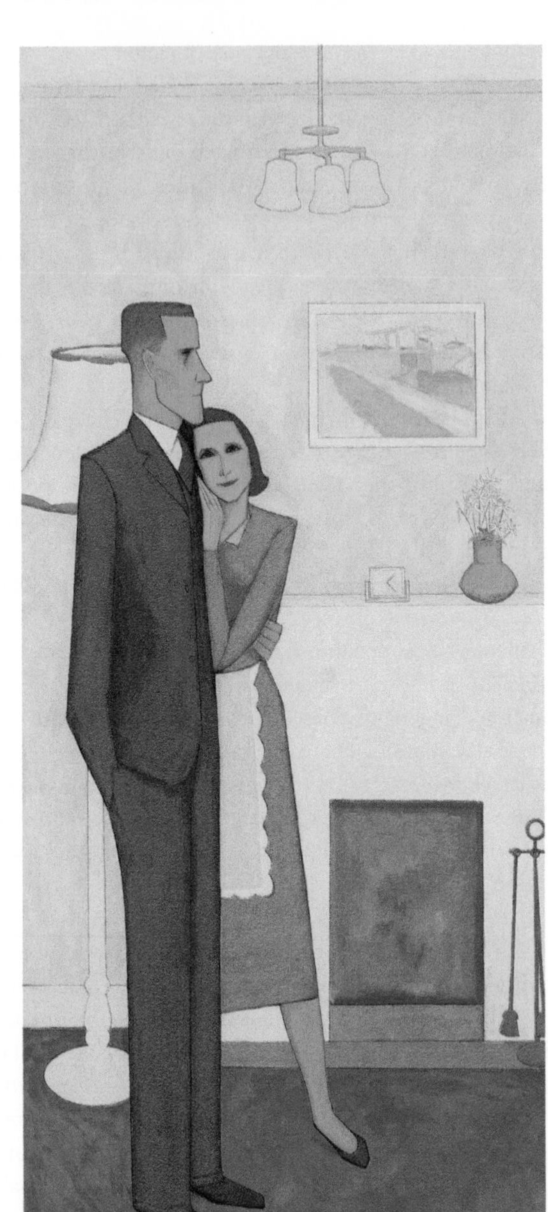

FIGURE 8.5 John Brack (Australia, b. 1920, d. 1999), *The New House* (1953), oil on canvas on hardboard, 142.5 x 71.2 cm.
Art Gallery of New South Wales, Australia, purchased with funds provided by the Gleeson O'Keefe Foundation 2013, © Helen Brack. Photo by AGNSW, Jenni Carter 192.2013.

The husband in *The New House* is ramrod straight, a pillar. He has a small, sour mouth, a caricature cartoon-hero clenched jaw and a puffed-out tie. He has important things on his mind (the mortgage perhaps, the knowledge of man's deep inhumanity to man, and, following the war, the fleeting nature of a life). He has a possessive hand wrapped around his wife's waist. She is his, along with the house; she even matches the colours of the fire screen, the hearth rug (which will catch the sparks when the fire is burning) the brass fire-tools, the vase containing the perfumed flowers, while her apron is the colour of the wall-paper. Her eyes are a deep violet blue, blurred a little as if by tears, and they look straight out of the painting at the viewer. She curves her body around the upright pillar of her husband's strength. She brings life to him, she cherishes him, she will lose herself in her love for him while she simultaneously becomes a wife of the house.

Like Sackville-West's Lady Slane, in *All Passions Spent*: "a young woman in a white dress, so dutiful, so admirably trained, and so wild at heart" (1931: 215) she hides, even from herself, her longing for something more. Only after her husband's death, at the age of 88, does Lady Slane admit to the one who had seen that wildness, that she should have been a painter: "So you were an artist, were you, potentially? But being a woman, that had to go by the board. I see. Now I understand why you sometimes looked so tragic when your face was in repose. I remember looking at you and thinking, That is a woman whose heart is broken" (1931: 219).

When the gallery re-opened and I could visit the original painting of *The New House*, I was compelled by those intense blue eyes that followed me wherever I stood. The hand on his chest has a smudge on it that looks like accidental dirt that should surely have been cleaned off. Looking closer I discovered it was her wedding ring, and that it did not go all the way around her finger. The incomplete ring that looks like dirt, the bridge whose two sides are built to separate, and was later bombed, and those blue eyes tell a story of well-trained obedience to marriage that co-exists with an intense longing for something more.

I wonder how many women, actually, could tolerate moulding themselves into that shape, inside the new house, while still providing the light, the liveliness, the illusion of love. Her enormous task is to disappear into the fabric of the new house while creating for her husband the safe place he can depend on. My mother loved and hated *Nant Gwylan*. She loved to entertain there, to show off her grand house, and she loved that it signalled to her sisters that she had got the best catch. And she hated it for the servitude it had caught her up in. She too, after my father's death, when she was 77, told me about her wild passion for my Uncle Llewellyn.

My father had promised my mother, before they were wed, that domesticity would not be all there was. There would be an overseas trip for the birth of each child. That, of course, turned out to be impractical. Decades later, my mother had not tired of drawing attention to those unfulfilled promises.

Writing about my mother so many years after her death was an apprenticeship to signs. So many of the signs pointed to the possibility, even probability, that she had never loved my father: "Everything that teaches us something emits signs; hieroglyphs … the signs are specific and constitute the substance of one world or another" (Deleuze, 2000: 4). Until I began my research and writing, the signs that she had not ever loved my father, were not signs that could be deciphered, and the story was one that could never be told.

> The worlds are unified by their formation of sign systems emitted by persons, objects, substances; we discover no truth, we learn nothing except by deciphering and interpreting. But the plurality of worlds is such that these signs are not of the same kind, do not have the same way of appearing, do not allow themselves to be deciphered in the same manner, do not have an identical relation with their meaning.
>
> (Deleuze, 2000: 5)

I can assemble a convincing catalogue of signs that support my intuited insight – but Norma's story will go on unfolding long after I am no longer deciphering and interpreting its continuities and discontinuities, and no longer seeking out the conditions that made it possible. There can be no ultimate or definitive narration of her life.

And so...

We each become a particular organism; we mobilise systems of meaning that enable that organism to signify and be signified; and we are subjectified, becoming the "subject of the enunciation recoiled into a subject of the statement" (Deleuze and Guattari, 1987: 159). This is true for both researcher and researched. Life itself opens in the flow, the movement, in between. And what is past is yet to come. Opening ourselves as researchers to a life as it is, or has been, lived by another, is not to find something or someone already there, but to enter into flows and forces that are social, material and semiotic. It is to become part of a relational event, a movement in between, in which we extend ourselves and our capacity to recognise the other in all their emergent multiplicity and difference. It is to make cuts that bring things together, and that takes things apart. It demands a great deal of hard work to acquire knowledge we don't have, and it depends on an openness to the not-yet-known. And sometimes it relies on a flash of intuition that changes everything.

References

Barad, K. 2007. *Meeting the Universe Halfway*. Durham, NC/ London: Duke University Press.

Barad, K. 2010. Quantum entanglements and hauntological relations of inheritance: dis/continuities, spacetime enfoldings, and justice-to-come. *Derrida Today*, 3(2), 240–268.

Bergson, H. 1998. *Creative Evolution* (trans. A. Mitchell). Mineola, NY: Dover Publications Inc.

Boochani, B. 2018. *No Friend but the Mountains* (trans. O. Tofighian). Sydney, NSW: Pan Macmillan Australia.

Davies, B. 2019. *New Lives in an Old Land. Re-turning to the Colonisation of New South Wales through Stories of my Parents and their Ancestors*. Sydney, NSW: Ornithorhynchus Paradoxus Books.

Deleuze, G. 1991. *Bergsonism* (trans. H. Tomlinson and B. Habberjam). New York: Zone Books.
Deleuze, G. 1995. Breaking things open. In G. Deleuze. *Negotiations 1972–1990* (trans. M. Joughin). New York: Columbia University Press, 83–93.
Deleuze, G. 2000. *Proust and Signs. The Complete Text* (trans. R. Howard). Minneapolis, MN: University of Minnesota Press.
Deleuze, G. and Guattari, F. 1987. *A Thousand Plateaus. Capitalism and Schizophrenia* (trans. B. Massumi). Minneapolis, MN: University of Minnesota Press.
Manning, E. 2015. Artfulness. In Grusin, R. (ed.), *The Nonhuman Turn*. Minneapolis, MN: Minnesota Press, 45–79.
Nancy, J.-L. 2000. *Being Singular Plural* (trans. R. D. Richardson and A. E. O'Byrne). Stanford, CA: Stanford University Press.
Nancy, J.-L. 2007. *Listening* (trans. C. Mandell). New York: Fordham University Press.
Oppenheimer, J. and Mitchell, B. 1989. *An Australian Clan: The Nivisons of New England*. Kenthurst, NSW: Kangaroo Press.
Sackville-West, V. 1931. *All Passions Spent*. London: Virago Press.
Wyatt, J. 2019. *Therapy, Stand-up, and the Gesture of Writing*. New York: Routledge.

9

ETHICO-ONTO-EPISTEMOLOGY

Inventing new possibilities of life

In which I explore the broad philosophical framework in which we might think about the onto-epistemology of a new materialist ethics. New materialism invites a profound re-thinking of what it is to be human/more-than human, and what our response-abilities are, in relation to each other, and to our nonhuman and earth others. I elaborate a set of twelve challenges for thinking-doing ethical research, drawing in particular on Deleuze and Barad, and Bennett.

Throughout this book I have explored the ways in which new materialist ethics is both ontological and epistemological. A new materialist ethics recognises that "[t]he material and the discursive are mutually implicated", and that they intra-act with each other, affecting each other (Barad, 2003: 812). Any assemblage "in its multiplicity, necessarily acts on semiotic flows, material flows, and social flows simultaneously" (Deleuze and Guattari, 1987: 22–23). Lying at the heart of new materialism is the insight that we are *of* the world rather than *in* it; we are intricately entangled in the world's becoming. We are more-than-human. We are less than we thought we were and much more. And we are emergent, entangled in the world's becoming. The very matter of the world, including human matter, lies in its ability to respond, and so responsibility lies at the heart of doing new materialist inquiry. Here, in this final chapter, I turn to the multiple challenges that such an ethics faces us with.

The *ontology* of ethics is micro and macro; it works on and in and between bodies, human and more-than-human, animate and inanimate. It works through institutional practices and habituated, normative practices. It involves the planet and its survivability. *Epistemologically* ethics is particularly interested in categorisations, and in the work they do, and in related acts of recognition and dis-recognition. Our repetitions and refrains are an entanglement of ontology and epistemology. Language is no longer thought of as a transparent tool with which to represent a world separate from us; it is, rather, a powerful agent that intra-acts with us and with the world.

To understand ethics in this way requires a great deal of erasing, clearing, flattening and shredding of standardised, institutionalised ethics:

> the painter does not paint on an empty canvas, and neither does the writer write on a blank page; but the page or canvas is already so covered with pre-existing, preestablished clichés that it is first necessary to erase, to clean, to flatten, even to shred, so as to let in a breath of air from the chaos that brings us the vision.
>
> (Deleuze and Guattari, 1994: 204)

The concept of ethics has been territorialised and re-territorialised through the dominance of royal-legal research, that has flourished under neoliberal modes of government. Sitting at the neoliberal heart of royal-legal ethics is the manipulation and control of the individualised, pathologised research participants, both researcher and researched. Neoliberalism is an extreme form of capitalism, which works to separate us off from each other and from the planet, and it turns us into obedient servants of capital. We have become hyper-competitive in the interests of survival, competing to produce what capital thinks it wants. We have learned to treat each other, and the Earth and its nonhuman inhabitants, as resources to exploit in the interests of our own survival and ascendance. Since around the 1990s we have been caught in institutional webs of control whose ostensible purpose is to increase national competitiveness through the intensification of productivity. Within the university sector this has manifested itself in a desire to bring academics under control. The tendency of academics to question any form of imposed order has been defined as a problem rather than a necessary (if sometimes irritating) virtue (Davies, 2019).

Neoliberal ethics presumes a social hierarchy in which the subjects of our research are weak and vulnerable, while we are characterised by an exploitative drive that has to be 'managed' by the legalistic mechanisms of 'ethics'. Such mechanisms are oblivious to the constitutive force of the mechanisms themselves, and the assumptions they hold in place. The royal-legal assemblage of ethics reduces the subjects of our research to being objects of the researcher's gaze. Their irreducible alterity, their difference, is set in place by the categorisation of them as *this* kind of person from *that* kind of background. Such categorisations place the Other as discrete and distinct from the self of the researcher, with the difference lying in the Other.

> Badiou poses an ethic of truths, as an alternative to contemporary ethics. An ethic of truths does not work from categorical difference, but similar to a Deleuzian process of differenciation, is an active process of opening oneself and others to the not-yet-known. This ethic of truths is situated and specific, focused on *events*, on happenings, which implicate everyone
>
> (Wyatt and Davies, 2011: 108)

New materialist ethics, and in Badiou's (2002) term, an ethic of truths, invites a collective knowing in being that "brings into play within us and outside us populations, multiplicities, territories, becomings, affects, events" (Deleuze and Parnet, 1987: 51). Contrary to neoliberal ethics, the subject who researches and the object of that research are not separate, with the researchers dominant and active, and the subjects subordinate and passive. The subjects of our research are not powerless "others", needing to be separated from us and protected from us.

What will count as research worth funding, and worth publishing, however, lies very often in the hands of neoliberalised rule-followers, rather than active, ambulatory researchers, though even ambulatory researchers can be seduced by the power of the royal-legal apparatuses of control. Being articulate, then, about what new materialism is and does, is of vital importance in the face of inevitable resistance from those apparatuses to the not-yet-known – which is where new materialist research dares to take itself.

Drawing on a reading of Hume, Deleuze pondered on the "problem of society" – how we understand it, how we make it work. One of the first issues he addresses is the obsession that has burgeoned, since the 1950s, with individuality and rights, and with the practices of categorisation that pit smaller and less powerful groups against the imagined whole. Deleuze defines the problem not as the individualisation itself, but as the reduction of our humanity that individualisation produces, which limits our capacity for sympathy: "The problem is no longer how to limit egotisms and the corresponding natural rights but how to go beyond partialities, how to pass from a 'limited sympathy' to an 'extended generosity,' how to stretch passions and give them an extension that they don't have on their own" (Deleuze, 2001: 46).

I touched on this challenge of movement from limited sympathy to extended generosity in my encounter with Rory (see Chapter 6), my encounter with the Holly Oak in Chapter 7, and my encounters with ancestors in Chapter 8. Extending our sympathies beyond what we already know, and becoming aware of our "shared vital materiality" (Bennett, 2010: 14) is integral to our, and to our planet's, survivability. Bennett admits that this "newfound attentiveness to matter and its powers will not solve the problem of human exploitation or oppression," but rather, she suggests, "it can inspire a greater sense of the extent to which all bodies are kin in the sense of [being] inextricably enmeshed in a dense network of relations" (Bennett, 2010: 12–13). In the face of that newfound attentiveness and our entanglement with each other and with our earth others, Barad argues in the same vein that ethics is about "entangled materializations" and our ability to respond:

> Ethics is ... not about right responses to a radically exteriorized other, but about responsibility and accountability for the lively relationalities of becoming, of which we are a part. Ethics is about mattering, about taking account of the entangled materializations of which we are part, including new configurations, new subjectivities, new possibilities. Even the smallest cuts matter. Responsibility is then a matter of the ability to respond. *Listening for the*

> *response of the other and an obligation to be responsive to the other, who is not entirely separate from what we call the self.*
>
> (Barad, 2011: 69; emphasis added)

Barad argues that researchers cannot be separated from their research questions, their language, their participants, and their own embodied selves. They are intra-actively emergent *with* them.

Neoliberalism has individualised us, and pitted individuals against each other in precarious, competitive social and institutional environments. The effect of that individualisation has been played out vividly in supermarkets during the pandemic, as dominant individuals pushed weaker individuals aside, or even started brawling with them, in irrational competition over items that have suddenly developed an equally irrational scarcity value, such as toilet paper and tinned tomatoes. It is an ugly version of humanity that has been encouraged to flourish in the service of strong economies. Quite wonderfully, in contrast, there are humans with conscience, who care for others: the firefighters here in the south-east of Australia, where fires ravaged the land and all its inhabitants; and now the health workers, globally, in the face of coronavirus.

Let me turn then to the twelve major challenges for ethical research.

1 *The first major challenge for ethical research is to disrupt the neoliberal, individualising limitations we have learned to enact in our dealings with human, animal and earth others. A new materialist ethics asks of us that we extend our capacity for generosity and response-ability.*

According to Deleuze (2001) philosophers have not operated separately from extreme capitalism and its depredations. Prior to the advent of neoliberalism, philosophers positioned themselves as isolated, moralising god-figures, who contemplated humanity as if it were separate from themselves. These god-figures, not unlike Catholic priests prior to the revelations of their sexual excesses, were the carriers of higher values. It was a powerful position and one that lingers among social and human scientists even now. Penn, for example, writes in 2020:

> The terms *observation* and *documentation* in the social sciences imply looking objectively from a position outside the event. Documentation, particularly via field notes, photography, video recording, or audio recording, further removes the researcher from the event in that an instrument or device, whether pencil, paper, camera, video camera, etc., intercedes between researcher and event ... Documentation, formalization, and systematicity in qualitative research have become signifiers of a rigorous empirical research practice.
>
> (Penn, 2020: 180)

Penn found herself in the god position as she held the video camera, torn between being response-able and remaining separate and objective and rigorous, not wanting to interfere with the recording of reality. Her research subject was Lionel, a 6-year-old boy who is being filmed while he is drawing:

> *He looks at the video camera and then around the camera at me, "Can you please help me spell baa?" Though I'm still recording, I can't ignore a direct request for help. I mouth "Ba ... ah ..." He repeats "Ba ... aaaaaah," frowns, taps his pencil. He carefully writes one letter and looks up again, anxiety etched on his face. "Ch ... ba ... ka ...U? U?" I have a difficult time remaining neutral and unengaged but tell him, "I can't help you when I'm filming. You can do it."*
>
> (Penn, 2020: 180)

The drawing that Lionel was struggling with, was of a strong soldier shooting someone much smaller than himself, with threatening machines flying above them. He writes underneath that both are strong. Penn is left with ethical questions about her choice not to help a boy clearly in despair, which she cannot easily resolve other than by attributing agency to the video camera with its apparent desire (as she imagines it) for uncontaminated reality.

For the philosophers, when the god-position they had adopted came increasingly under fire, they took up the position of moral legislators who carried and preserved the higher values. In the altercation between the fictional characters, Sano and Enfermada, in my much-cited positioning paper (Davies and Harré, 1990), Sano was a philosopher who held very firmly to his position of moral ascendance, and with it his power to know what the higher values were, and to manifest them. To be challenged by a feminist upstart (who was, after all, only a woman, and a colonial, even worse, a rural colonial) was intolerable to him.

Deleuze argues that both the god-position and the moral legislator position are harmful in their intransigence, and in their presumption of a justifiable elevation above those others, human and nonhuman, who they constituted as their inferiors. What he argues for is a further shift toward poetry and creativity: "*To create is to lighten, to unburden life, to invent new possibilities of life*" (Deleuze, 2001: 69; emphasis added).

Those new forms of creativity and invention require the capacity for sympathy, and openness to being transported outside existing certainties. Our duration, as human, entangled with others, human, animal and earth others, "means invention, the creation of forms, the continual elaboration of the absolutely new" (Bergson, 1998: 11). Furthermore, to endure, Bennett (2010: xiv) argues, we need to cultivate "patient, sensory attentiveness to nonhuman forces operating outside and inside the human body".

2 *The second challenge for ethical research is to stop placing ourselves above the subjects we research, as the holders of "higher values", with the right to judge others. Instead of carrying the burden of upholding those conservative values we must rediscover how to become creators, who work towards new possibilities of life in interdependent relations with others.*

Deleuze's (2001) reflections on Nietzsche open up a way of thinking about this question further – about what our limitations have been in our ways of thinking about, and of relating to, others. He begins with thinking about nihilism and the death of God: "man makes himself even more ugly when, no longer in need of an external authority, he denies himself what was denied him and spontaneously takes on the policing and the burdens that he no longer thinks come from the outside" (Deleuze, 2001: 72).

It is interesting to link these reflections to the many forms of violence that proliferate globally, both among individuals and systemically from governing bodies. Among individuals, for example, violence against women is soaring, particularly during the pandemic. Governmental violence is also increasing, globally, in the quest, for example, to quell dissidents and punish outsiders; governments condone unspeakable forms of torture, not just in the name of war, which is bad enough, and not just of adults deemed to be enemies of the state, but of children, of people seeking refuge, of people who dare to dissent and of people who are "not like us". In Australia, for example, the federal government, enthralled by Trump, treats investigative journalists as enemies of the state.

3 *The third challenge for ethical research is to become aware of, and open up alternatives to, the onto-epistemological forms of ugliness that human behaviour can sink into through the individualisation and commercialisation of policing and punishment. Ethical research must work to make visible, and to comprehend the forces and powers of the assemblages through which individuals are violated, where the social flows in between are devoid of sympathy and response-ability.*

Being open to the other is enlivening, taking us outside our familiar modes of categorisation, and into an emergent being-becoming. Such openness to difference and to differenciation is a prerequisite for tuning into the biosphere we co-inhabit. Moral judgement, in contrast, is a self-protective measure that places a barrier between the one who judges and the one who is judged. Our task, as researchers, is to seek "the enveloped modes of existence" (Deleuze 1980: np) through which life is made, and through which life endures.

The art of being non-judgemental must extend to ourselves, emergent within the research. Judgements of guilt and innocence are not the point. The point is to develop our vestigial skills of sympathy and response-ability.

Deleuze elaborates Nietszche's stages of the triumph of nihilism:

1 *Resentment*: It's your fault ... it's your fault ... It's your fault if I'm weak and unhappy ... life itself is accused, separated from its power, separated from what it can do...
2 *Bad conscience*: It's my fault ... They interiorize the fault, say they are guilty, turn against themselves. But in this way, they set an example, they invite all of life to come and join them, they acquire a maximum of contagious power – they form reactive communities...

3 *The ascetic ideal*: The moment of sublimation. What the weak or reactive life ultimately wants is the negation of life. *Its* will to power is a will to nothingness, as a condition of its triumph…

4 *The death of God*: Nothing has changed, for the same reactive life, the same slavery [to so-called higher values] that had triumphed in the shadow of divine values now triumphs through human ones...

5 *The last man and the man who wants to die* … Following the higher men there arises the last man, the one who says: all is vain, better to fade away passively! [This end point] inspires in man the wish to actively destroy himself. (Deleuze, 2001: 78–82)

Turning from this ultimate point of nihilism, Nietzsche turned to affirmation: "Affirmation is the highest power of the will. But what is affirmed? The earth, life … what is affirmed is the One of multiplicity, the Being of becoming" (Deleuze 2001: 86–87).

In turning to and affirming life as multiple and emergent, we are enveloped not in a pre-planned order, but a world of serendipity, of surprises, not always comfortable, where the emergence of the new forces thought to open itself to what it does not yet know. That unpredictability brings with it a heightened responsibility for what is being made to matter.

4 *The fourth challenge, then, is to recognise the undesirability of attempts to control the future, through, for example, detailed research plans from which we may not deviate, and conceptual apparatuses which dictate how our research must progress. Being open to the not yet known requires being open to being surprised, open to chance, and to the unexpected – these are the* sine qua non *of creativity.*

In Barad's philosophy, creativity and response-ability are central; her primary interest is in the ways in which things come to matter. Individuals no longer float free of discourse, or morality, or the earth; they are epistemologically, ontologically and ethically entangled with each other and with the matter of the earth:

> [Justice entails] the ongoing practice of being open and alive to each meeting, each intra-action, so that we might use our ability to respond, our responsibility, to help awaken, to breathe life into ever new possibilities for living justly. The world and its possibilities for becoming are remade in each meeting. *How then shall we understand our role in helping constitute who and what come to matter?*
>
> (Barad 2007, x; emphasis added)

5 *The fifth challenge for ethical research is to remain cognisant of and responsive to the intra-action between the territorialising, stabilising forces and the vitality of playful, poetic disruptions. Justice cannot be generated solely by laws and law-enforcement – justice is emergent in every moment, and in every movement in between.*

What contemporary, institutionalised ethics fails to see, from a Baradian perspective, is that we are necessarily *entangled* in the events we study, and that this is not some form of mistake to be corrected. Both researchers and researched are sentient, relational beings who affect and are open to being affected in their intra-actions with others. In a new materialist ethics, we are responsible for what it is that is being made to matter in the questions we ask, the methods we use, the encounters we engage in, and in the thinking, the writing and art-making that we engage in and experiment with. There is no single mo(ve)ment we might find ourselves immersed in that does not require of us to ask what it is that is being made to matter, and *how* it is being made to matter. It is never just oneself as a researcher intra-acting with a research subject. All of us are entangled in complex systems. We are responsible collectively, materially and epistemologically. We cannot refuse responsibility for what we believe and what we do – or for what is generally believed and generally done. Our responsibility is both macro and micro, systemic and intimate. Machines may be granted power, as Penn did with her video machine, but that does not mean it is ethical to give precedence to that power or to leave it unacknowledged. "Ethicality," Barad writes, "entails hospitality to the stranger threaded through oneself and through all being and non/being" (Barad, 2015: 163).

Our collectivity is not just human collectivity. The nonhuman is integral to our existence: "animals, plants, organisms, climatic systems, technologies, or ecosystems" (Grusin, 2015: x) are all at play in ways that the conventional dominance of human subjects has made us blind to: "feeling, desiring and experiencing are not singular characteristics or capacities of human consciousness. Matter feels, converses, suffers, desires, yearns and remembers" (Barad, 2011: 59).

6 *The sixth challenge is to be open, and respond creatively, to the nonhuman animal and earth others, and to the more-than-human of ourselves.*

Both human and non- or more-than-human intra-act within events that are affecting them and being affected by them: "Different material intra-actions produce different materialisations of the world and hence there are specific stakes in how responsiveness is enacted. In an important sense, it matters to the world how the world comes to matter" (Barad, 2008: 332). If we find ourselves intra-acting with concepts and/or apparatuses that demand inhumane behaviour, we are responsible for generating new possibilities:

7 *The seventh challenge, in Barad's words: "is about accounting for our part of the entangled webs we weave… [and] the entangled materialisations we help enact and are a part of bringing about, including new configurations, new subjectivities, new possibilities – even the smallest cuts matter" (Barad, 2008: 335–336; emphasis added).*

An ethics that is committed to inventing new possibilities for life re-engages with the desire for, and belief in, the possibility of a more just world, while acknowledging that, globally, justice is probably as rare now as it ever has been, if not more so.

It is vitally important that we make an account of our part in what is being brought about as we seek to create new possibilities.

In making such an account, we can't take up any of the dominant, well-practised, liberal–humanist refrains in which we position ourselves as looking out for others less fortunate than ourselves. It can't be accomplished by an explicit or implicit claim of oneself as a being who is coherent and lucid, superior to the mystery of the others who are to be researched, revealed, and helped. The aim of ethical research can no longer be the engineering of an ideal ethical future in which we will have eliminated injustice. Our "virtue" in new materialist research is much more challenging than that.

It has been common practice, particularly since the end of the Second World War, to turn to regulation and to the law to bring about a just world. Beginning with *The Universal Declaration of Human Rights*, for example, some sought to make the entire world a place where gross violations, such as those committed by the Nazis and the Stasi, would become inconceivable. Those who violated the ideals of humanity and justice would have to answer for themselves in court. *The Declaration* asserted, for example that no one would be subjected to torture or to cruel, inhuman or degrading treatment or punishment (*Article 5*), and that everyone would have the right to seek and to enjoy in other countries asylum from persecution (*Article 14*).

Australia signed the declaration, and, as a signatory, is legally obliged to follow it, or face public condemnation. The Australian government confidently passes moral judgement on other nations when they fail to live up to the *Declaration*'s principles, unless, of course, it is a nation, such as the USA, on whom it is dependent economically or militarily. When it does pass judgement, it does so, astonishingly, as if its own record is clean. It incarcerates and tortures indigenous children, it tortures people seeking asylum in privatised off-shore detention centres, whose diabolical practices have been kept secret, as have Australian activities on the water between Australia and Indonesia, where refugees' boats are "turned back" (Macken, 2019). Black lives are repeatedly destroyed by the very people assigned to keep them safe. The aged are denied medical treatment and locked in to die during the pandemic. Children are sexually assaulted. A list of atrocities that could go on and on.

How are we to make sense of this profound schism in the meaning of "human"? To be humane we understand as an unqualified good. Yet humans are capable of extreme brutality, not just in the past, and not just from individual "bad eggs", or from the wild ones and trouble-makers – but humanity in general, throughout spacetime as we know it, engages in individual and institutional brutality.

Barad asks an extraordinary and provocative question based on quantum field theory. At the heart of ourselves, in the matter of ourselves, is matter that she calls inhuman matter. Perhaps what we need to do she suggests, is face that inhumanity that lies in all of us: "*What if it is only in facing the inhuman – the indeterminate non/being non/becoming of mattering and not mattering* – that an ethics committed to the rupture of indifference can arise?" (Barad, 2015: 161–162).

8 *The eighth challenge is to overcome indifference and to develop compassion. The weight of this challenge is difficult to grasp after generations of liberal humanist individualism. Our common humanity is not an abstract idea in new materialism, about how bodies might, in an ideal world, relate to each other, but the immediacy of compassion – of thinking, feeling and responding in the now.*

One of the classrooms I studied some decades ago was that of "Mr Good" (Davies, 1990, 1994). Mr Good was so popular and so successful in working with children who had fallen foul of the school system, that his class was de-zoned; parents from anywhere in the city could apply to have their child in his classroom on the basis of their child's unhappiness in, or disaffection from, the school system.

Mr Good designed individual learning programmes for each child. His classroom had the look of an industrious beehive, each "bee" knowing what it was doing, quietly communicating whenever necessary with the other bees, and busily getting on with its own tasks, moving from one place to another in the classroom. In one of the group interviews with the children, when I asked them what they liked best about being in Mr Good's class, they said "When he says: 'Still as that!'"

When Mr Good wanted to address all the children at once, he would hold his finger in the air in the midst of his busy beehive, and would say quietly, "Still as that". The children would each freeze in whatever bodily posture they were in at that very moment – whether mid-stride or half-way to sitting down, or immersed in solving a maths problem, and they would listen attentively while he spoke. When he finished speaking, and put his finger down, they would unfreeze, and go happily back to work.

Mr Good had found a way to pay attention to the singularity and desire of each child, and at the same time to bring them together as one listening, playful organism, taking pleasure in being together as one (the "One of multiplicity, the Being of becoming", Deleuze, 2001: 86–7). My own teacher education students at the time of this study (notoriously anxious about being able to control a class full of children) expressed disbelief when they saw the video I had made of the 'still-as-that' moment. "He must have secretly thrashed them," one doubting Thomas surmised. But no, existing in a moment of commonly experienced humanity was, it seemed, highly pleasurable in itself. Children who had been chronic bed-wetters, and school truants, were now happy to be at school, each confident in developing their own direction without interfering in the direction of others, while taking pleasure in being part of a creative collective.

"Still as that" was a visible, audible, playful call together of that multiplicity and difference into a common humanity.

While we understand that animals can move together in complex harmony with each other – bees managing their beehives while roving over vast distances, for example, or butterflies staging mass migrations that take several generations to complete, we find it much more difficult to think of ourselves being/becoming within the collective. Our individualism, and in particular our heightened individualism under neoliberal regimes, blinds us to the extent we are actually emergent within collectives, and that includes neoliberal collectives. In observing animals (including the animal within ourselves) it is possible to see our collectivity as extraordinary and beautiful, and, potentially, as devastatingly destructive.

The state department of education initially refused to promote Mr Good, as his teaching practices did not fit precisely within their guidelines. My students and I made a video tape of his classroom, with parts of the interview with him and the interviews with the children spliced in. Mr Good submitted the video to the departmental appeals committee, and he won his appeal. We had recorded his lines of flight, his ambulatory methods, his compassion, and rendered them comprehensible within the assemblage of the state school system.

Because the nature of matter, the matter that connects all of us, human, animal and earth, is emergent, relational and entangled, justice can never be a settled state of affairs. It is necessarily ongoing, which is why our response-ability matters so much. What we can become is a matter of our entanglements, which are much larger than ourselves. How we touch others, and are touched, lies at the heart of responsibility:

> [A]ll material "entities," are entangled relations of becoming, there is also the fact that materiality "itself" is always already touched by and touching infinite configurings of other beings and other times ... Each of "us" is constituted in response-ability. Each of "us" is constituted as responsible for the other, as being in touch with the other.
>
> (Barad, 2015: 160–161)

Barad makes, at the same time, a very strong plea for the importance of thinking, and of experimenting with new ways of thinking and doing both life itself, and research. She does not advocate a random spinning off in any direction, but the hard work of thinking, and a collaborative touching, involving all the senses, a human/nonhuman touching which enables response-ability:

> Spinning off in any direction is neither theorizing nor viable; it loses the thread, the touch of entangled beings (be)coming together/apart. All life forms (including inanimate forms of liveliness) do theory. The idea is to do collaborative research, to be in touch, in ways that enable response-ability.
>
> (Barad, 2015: 155)

It is in thinking about touch as vital to both human and nonhuman existence, with our own inhumanity being integral to that concept, that Barad's argument takes on its greatest power.

9 *And so to the ninth challenge: it is in becoming vulnerable to the other – in a positive sense of vulnerability, meaning openness – that justice can begin: "The sense of exposure to the other is crucial and so is the binding obligation that is our vulnerability, our openness"* (Barad, 2015: 162).

Rather than being individual agents capable of bringing about the necessary changes in systems external to ourselves, we are emergent beings caught up in the "intra-active becoming of the world": "Responsibility entails an ongoing responsiveness to the entanglement of self and other, here and there, now and then" (Barad, 2007: 394). In this new thinking about justice, enacting a just world is not an ideal to be realised at some future time and place but a moment by moment accomplishment of just ways of knowing in being in all our intra-actions.

We are each entangled in a world in flux, a world made up of multiple competing forces – not individual agents of change, but agents whose actions and thoughts *matter*. Justice in this iteration of it involves us in thoughts and actions that are both macro-political, challenging established structures and identities, and micro-political – generating, through new ways of thinking, new actions, new lines of flight, molecular becomings, which open escape-routes from familiar refrains, from established patterns and coherences.

There is no simple method to arrive at these new ways of thinking and doing research. We rely on some well-known practices, such as interviewing and observation, but we must jettison much of the conceptual baggage that has attended them, baggage often carrying with it the imprint of logical positivism that has not been thoroughly wiped, shredded and cleared out of the way. One moves rhizomatically (Deleuze) or diffractively (Barad) in the hope of generating new and ethical ways of knowing in being that are not trapped inside old binaries. But how is this to be done? Grosz (2011: 75) asks:

> How can we produce knowledges, techniques, methods, practices that bring out the best in ourselves, that open us up to the embrace of an unknown and open-ended future, that bring into existence new kinds of beings, new kinds of subjects, and new relations to objects?

In Deleuzian terms the challenge is to move beyond thinking and acting difference as categorical difference, toward thinking and acting as differenciation – to becoming, and going on becoming other than we were. We are of the world and the world "is made up of modifications, disturbances, changes of tension and of energy, and nothing else" (Deleuze, 1991: 76). For Barad it is about keeping thought alive and emergent, "being responsible and responsive to the world's patternings and murmurings … being open to the world's aliveness, allowing oneself to be lured by curiosity, surprise, and wonder" (Barad, 2015: 154).

Our work as new materialist researchers is to attune ourselves to our entanglements with human, nonhuman and earth others, to develop strategies, conceptual and practical, through which we can imagine and enact the world differently. For Deleuze, that attuning is not about "the interiority of a sovereign subject" but about "the spaces that connect all of us to one another and to the world we inhabit" (Stark, 2017: 111). Justice in the thinking/doing of it demands openness to the other, to difference, to what we don't know. It demands of us that we find new ways of connecting with the world, human, nonhuman, more-than-human, which involves giving up on our own fixities.

Neoliberal technologies have made us goal oriented and risk averse, our survival depending on satisfying institutional measures of success – all of them tied to productivity – rather than to the production of "knowledges, techniques, methods, practices that bring out the best in ourselves" (Grosz, 2011: 75). We are pressed into the production of measurable institutionally approved objects. Without even being aware of it, we are at risk of ignoring the harm that we become party to in the interests of our own enduring, and individualised surviving.

As new materialist researchers, teachers, colleagues, activists, we do not begin with the end-point – the products – but in the middle of life's events in which we are emergent beings, open to "the embrace of an unknown and open-ended future" (Grosz, 2011: 75).

10 *Our tenth challenge is to ask how our responses, and our accounts of the world we encounter, shape the world that is to come? "What's at stake" in those responses and those accounts, Nancy says, is the work of making and re-making the world. He suggests that we consider, in the execution of our research, this advice: "Act as if the maxim of your action were to become a universal law of nature" (Nancy, 2017: 27; paraphrasing Kant).*

In making the world that is to come, the quality of attention matters. And this brings me to the eleventh challenge:

11 *Our eleventh challenge is to bring a quality of attention to each moment, each movement, each thought, each event, and each act of writing, that takes us outside ourselves and into the becoming of new entanglements.*

The singularities of being and becoming that we generate, both through our technical expertise and through our quality of attention, takes us elsewhere, and to new entangled becomings. Nancy explores that singularity and emergent being in the dissolving of boundaries between listener and sound, where the listener becomes indissociable from the music, and where both listener and music become other than themselves. It is the *entanglement itself*, rather than the two separate entities, he suggests, that resonates:

> To be listening is thus to enter into tension and to be on the lookout for a relation to self: not, it should be emphasized, a relationship to "me" (the supposedly given subject), or the "self" of the other (the speaker, the musician, also supposedly given, with his subjectivity), but to the relationship in self, so to speak, as it forms a "self" or a "to itself" in general … [where] "self" is precisely nothing available (substantial or subsistent) to which one can be "present," but precisely the resonance of a return [renvoi] … listening – the opening stretched toward the register of the sonorous … not as a metaphor for access to self, but as the reality of this access, reality consequently indissociably "mine" and "other," "singular" and "plural," as much as it is "material" and spiritual and "signifying" and "a-signifying."
>
> (Nancy, 2007: 12)

This quality of attention to an encounter with the other is not rooted in moral judgements of self and other, of self separate from the other. It begins with the proposition that we are all *of* the world, and thus of the same matter, and at the same time multiplicative and endlessly divergent. Life, in this understanding of it is motion, and its capacity to endure depends on the emergence of the new.

Emergent listening mobilises all our senses (Davies, 2014) and immerses us in emergent multiplicities. It takes both stillness and perseverance. Stillness "allows other 'planes' of reality to be perceivable" (O'Sullivan, 2001: 127). We open up the possibility of "an engagement with that which goes beyond premature observations and preconceived neutralizing facts" (Manning, 2015: 63). Perseverance involves us in multiple provocations to thought, in a dogged hanging out with what we don't yet know how to think. Research, Manning (2015: 48) observes, is "a rigorous process that consists in pushing technique to its limits, revealing its technicity – the very outdoing of technique that makes the more-than of experience felt. Bergson calls it a long encounter, a mode of work, that has nothing to do with synthesis or recognition". It is artful creating of "an opening to the unsayable, the unthinkable. And sympathy for the force of this unthinkability" (Manning, 2015: 64). It resists codifying experiences, one's own and the other's, and it resists sorting experiences into existing categories of meaning. It draws on imagination to go beyond the limits of the already known: "it is up to the imagination to reflect passion, to make it resonate and go beyond the limits of its natural partiality and presentness" (Deleuze, 2001: 48). It involves encounters with the other, both human and more-than-human, and asks of them "*How is this possible*... Which manner of Being does this imply" (Deleuze, 1980: np).

12 Which brings me to our final challenge: to open up the unsayable and the unthinkable.

We are living, as it happens, in a time when our capacity to encompass the new is stretched to the limit – in Australia, with the multiple devastations of long-term drought followed by fires of an intensity never seen before in recent history. In the 2019–20 fires, 2,439 homes were lost; more than a billion animals were killed nationally, with 800 million in NSW alone. Twenty-one per cent of Australian temperate broadleaf and mixed forests were burnt, well above the annual average of around 2 per cent. The bushfires are estimated to have spewed more carbon dioxide into the atmosphere than Australia's annual emissions, of around 531 million tonnes. The emissions from the fires are estimated at between 650 million and 1.2 billion tonnes, or about equivalent to the annual emissions from commercial aircraft worldwide, and more than Germany's annual emissions.

Those of us living in the city, out of the path of the fires, breathed the smoke and shut ourselves into our houses and apartments, and downloaded apps to find out how dangerous it was to breathe the air. The grit that managed to find its way inside my apartment's closed windows included large chunks. Whose body, I wondered, do the bits of grit come from as I wiped them up – as if they were dirt – yet it was others' lives and livelihoods, lives of people and animals, and trees and houses that covered the surfaces of my home, that now live inside my lungs and probably also in my bloodstream.

Before we had a chance to recover ourselves from the deadly fires, floods came, and then the pandemic, followed by global economic collapse. And while we are numb from the enormity of these changes, and the foreboding of the enormity to come with climate change, we are told to stay at home, to change our bodily habits, and to take up an unprecedented stillness and repetitiveness. We are asked to make time stand still while the world potentially collapses around us – unless, of course, we are counted by government as "essential"...

But change goes on, however minute the movements are. McGregor, for example, describes going to help friends clear the devastating mess from their fire-ravaged land:

> We are walking along a sandy trail that was once the only path, such was the thickness of the scrub. Now, through the skeletal black, the neighbours are visible. A market gardener who lost a shed full of tractors and his weatherboard house; a pastoral property whose house survived, situated as it is in the middle of a large paddock. An apiarist whose bees all died. At the bottom of the hill is a creek that feeds Bargo River, now in rare flow...
>
> All the species endemic to the area lived here. Gang-gang cockatoos, crimson rosellas, spinebills, honeyeaters. Stringybark, silvertop ash, bloodwood, grey and scribbly gums. Mountain devils, acacias, geebungs. Now the place is quiet. Ants have been busy – little mounds of ochre-coloured soil are everywhere underfoot – and there are new shoots of native grass and fungi, which digest carbon from the ash.
>
> (McGregor, 2020: 16)

And so...

Entanglement has threaded its way as a concept through all of these chapters. It confounds usual ways of thinking about causality; old linear trajectories give way to multiple lines of force that pin us down and give rise to disruptions, to re-turns, to mergings, and, now and then, to new thought. The lines of force are multiple, co-implicated, and always emergent. It confounds the concept of the individualised, autonomous self: "Intelligibility and materiality are not fixed aspects of the world, but rather intertwined agential performances" (Barad, 2008: 325). The concept of entanglement disrupts the taken-for-granted ascendancy of the human species, and it abandons the humanist version of what we are – moving from identities to emergent, singular multiplicities.

Humanism's subject assumes, even morally requires, dominance over itself, and it assumes self-righteous dominance over the other-than-human world. It configures itself as a causal agent, and it imagines itself to be its own cause. Here, in contrast, the post-humanist subject no longer lies at the centre of all meaning-making, and is no longer, collectively, the sole agent commanding the worlding of the world.

New materialist thinking proposes that all of us are enmeshed and entangled with each other in multiple becomings with the more-than-human world. We are "relentlessly becoming-with ... in unexpected collaborations and combinations, in hot compost piles. We become-with each other or not at all. That kind of material semiotics is always situated, someplace and not noplace, entangled and worldly" (Haraway, 2016: 4). Our stories, our bodies, our ethics, utter one another, as do the entangled systemic, strata on/in which our lives are embedded.

Re-thinking the matter of our place and our being/becoming in and of the world, involves coming to grips with our own material indeterminacy: "there are no separate isolated entities that can be observed from outside, 'entities' do not have a fixed inherent nature (wave or particle). Duality of wave and particle – and *indeterminacy more generally* – is inherent to matter. This indeterminacy is 'in' matter (or simply *is* matter)" (de Freitas, 2017: 743). This pulls the plug on that aspect of the humanist project in which we each seek to discover "who we are" as if our stories had the power to establish the truth of our "individual selves" – selves contained in our skin and fundamentally unavailable to each other. We are indeterminate, and yet, too, we hold on to our refrains, and with them our sense of continuity, of safety, of commitment. We hold on to our recognisable presence in case we slide into the wildness that Deleuze & Guattari (1987) warn us against.

This doubleness of vision, on the one hand where boundaries are dissolved, and on the other where we assemble ourselves as beings capable of acting response-ably, is challenging. I explore that doubleness in the collage with which I bring this odyssey to a close.

I began this art-work, intuitively, with the feathers, and with the portrait by Aurélie Petiot that I'd cut out of a magazine some time ago. It had been sitting waiting for me to do something with it. Because of the coronavirus lockdown I had to work with whatever material I had to hand. For a surface to work on I chose a painting of a wave I'd made in a workshop some years before. The image I had in mind, that had lived in my mind since the fires, was of burnt trees in a forest, now looking like upright burnt matches. My idea was to dissolve the boundaries between humans, forest and fire, and birds falling dead from the sky. When the trees became indistinguishable from the fire, I scraped their outline with the handle of the brush, and the wave underneath re-surfaced to line the trees with waterfalls of tears, that are remnants of waves. With those tears, and with a feather earring for Aurélie Petiot's Pre-Raphaelite portrait, the collage drew together my sorrow for the harm done to the earth, and for the birds falling dead in the heat of the flames. What began to emerge was a blurring of the boundary between the sorrowing woman and the burning forest. I sank into the image I had created; I wept tears of sympathy for the earth, and for the fragile futurity of the human species:

> Bergson calls the mechanism by which this future-feeling arises 'sympathy.' Sympathy not 'of' the human but 'with' experience in the making. 'We call intuition that sympathy by which we are transported to the interior of an object to coincide with what it has that is unique and, consequently, inexpressible.
>
> (Manning, 2015: 48–49, citing Lapoujade)

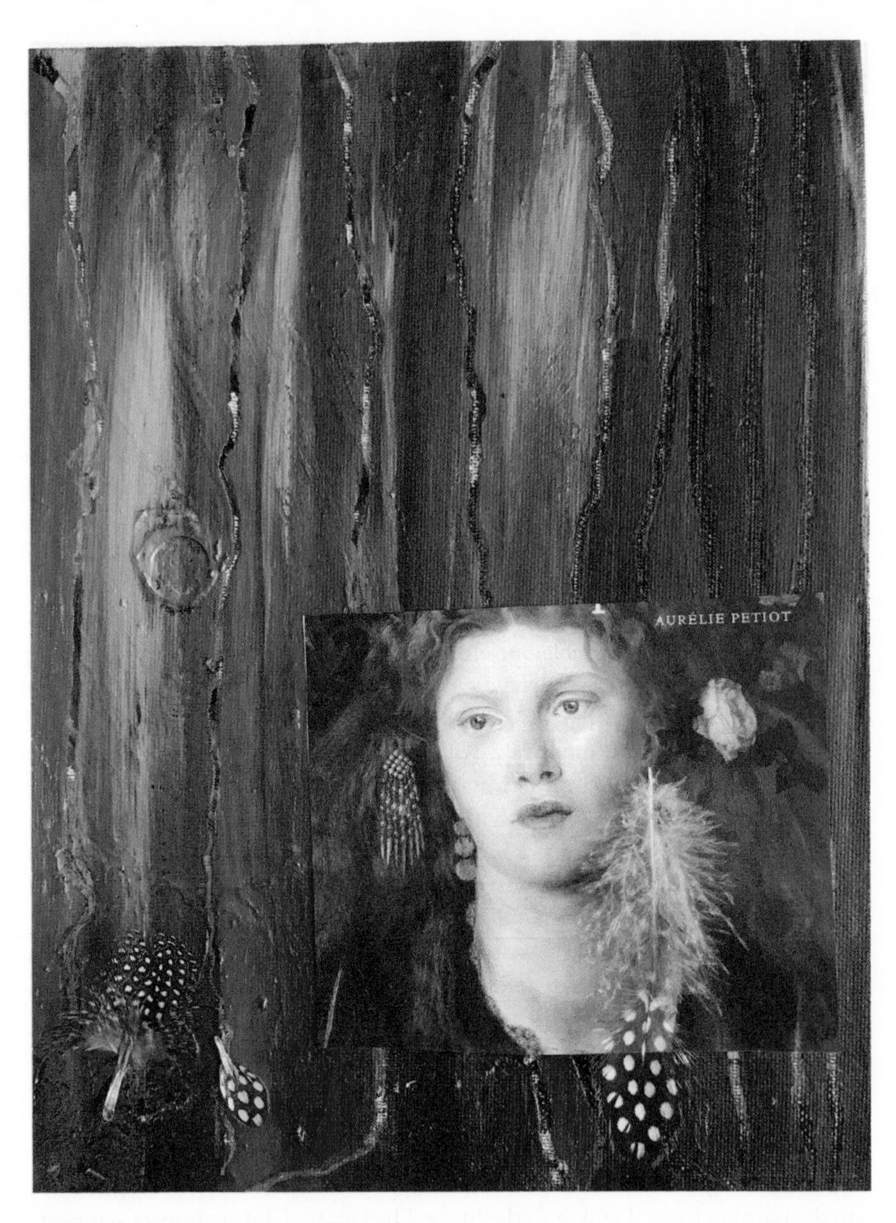

FIGURE 9.1 Bronwyn Davies, Sympathy.
Collage. Photograph of collage by Bronwyn Davies, 2020.

References

Badiou, A. 2002. *Ethics. An Essay on the Understanding of Evil* (trans. P. Hallward). London: Verso.

Barad, K. 2003. Posthumanist performativity: How matter comes to matter. *Signs: Journal of Women in Culture and Society*, 28(3), 801–831.

Barad, K. 2007. *Meeting the Universe Halfway*, Durham, NC/London: Duke University Press.

Barad, K. 2008. Queer causation and the ethics of mattering. In M. J. Hyrd and N. Giffney (eds), *Queering the Non/Human*. Taylor and Francis Group. ProQuest Ebook, 247–352.

Barad, K. 2011. Interview with Karen Barad. In R. Dolphijn and I. van der Tuin (eds), *New Materialism: Interviews and Cartographies*. Ann Arbor, MI: Open Humanities Press, 48–70.

Barad, K. 2015. On touching the inhuman that therefore I am (vo1. 1). In K. Stakemeier and S. Witzgall (eds), *Power of Material/Politics of Materiality*. Zurich, SW: Diaphanes, 153–164.

Bennett, J. 2010. *Vibrant matter. A Political Ecology of Things*. Durham, NC: Duke University Press.

Bergson, H. 1998. *Creative Evolution* (trans. A. Mitchell). Mineola, NY: Dover Publications Inc.

Davies, B. 1990. Agency as a form of discursive practice. A classroom scene observed. *British Journal of Sociology of Education*, 11(3), 341–361.

Davies, B. 1994. *Poststructuralist Theory and Classroom Practice*. Geelong, Vic: Deakin University Press.

Davies, B. 2014. *Listening to Children: Being and Becoming*. London: Routledge.

Davies, B. 2019. Life in neoliberal institutions: Australian stories. *Qualitative Inquiry*, 1–7. DOI:10.1177/10778004|9878737.

Davies, B. and Harré, R. 1990. Positioning: The discursive production of selves. *Journal for the Theory of Social Behaviour*, 20(1), 43–63.

de Freitas, E. 2017. Karen Barad's quantum ontology and posthuman ethics. Rethinking the concept of relationality. *Qualitative Inquiry*, 23(9), 741–748.

Deleuze, G. 1980. Cours Vincennes, 12/21/1980. http://www.webdeleuze.com/php/texte.php?cle=190andgroupe=Spinoza andlangue=2) (accessed 10 February 2010).

Deleuze, G. 1991. *Bergsonism* (trans. H. Tomlinson). New York: Zone Books.

Deleuze, G. 2001. Immanence: A life (trans. A. Boyman). In G. Deleuze (ed.), *Pure Immanence: Essays on a Life*. New York: Zone.

Deleuze, G. and Guattari, F. 1987. *A Thousand Plateaus. Capitalism and Schizophrenia*, (trans. B. Massumi). Minneapolis, MN: University of Minnesota Press.

Deleuze, G. and Guattari, F. 1994. *What Is Philosophy?* (trans. H. Tomlinson and G. Burchell). New York: Columbia University Press.

Deleuze, G. and Parnet, C. 1987. *Dialogues 11: Revised Edition* (trans. H. Tomlinson and B. Habberjam). New York: Columbia University Press.

Grosz, E. 2011. *Becoming Undone: Darwinian Reflections on Life, Politics and Art*. Durham, NC/London: Duke University Press.

Grusin, R. (ed.) 2015. *The Nonhuman Turn*. Minneapolis, MN: University of Minnesota Press.

Haraway, D. J. 2016. *Staying with the Trouble. Making Kin in the Chthulucene*. Durham, NC/London: Duke University Press.

Manning, E. 2015. Artfulness. In Grusin, R. (ed.), *The Nonhuman Turn*. Minneapolis, MN: Minnesota Press.

McGregor, F. 2020. Slow work. *The Monthly*, April. 15–17.

Macken, J. 2019. The melancholic torturer: How Australia became a nation that tortures refugees. *Journal of Sociology*, 56, 9–22.

Nancy, J.-L. 2007. *Listening* (trans. C. Mandell). New York, NY: Fordham University Press.

Nancy, J.-L. 2017. *The Possibility of a World: Conversations with Pierre-Philippe Jandin* (trans. T. Holloway and F. Méchain). New York: Fordham University Press.

O'Sullivan, S. 2001. The aesthetics of affect: Thinking art beyond representation. *Angelaki: Journal of Theoretical Humanities*, 6(3), 125–135.

Penn, L. R. 2020. Quantum ethics: Intra-actions in researching with children. In C. Schulte (ed.), *Ethics and Research with Young Children: New Perspectives*. London: Bloomsbury Academic, 173–187.

Stark, H. 2017. *Feminist Theory after Deleuze*. London: Bloomsbury Academic.

Wyatt, J. and Davies, B. 2011. Ethics. In Wyatt, J., Gale, K., Gannon, S. and Davies, B. *Deleuze and Collaborative Writing: An Immanent Plane of Composition*. New York: Peter Lang, 105–129.

AUTHOR INDEX

SUBJECT INDEX